Diagnosis and Management of Neck and Back Pain

IN PRIMARY CARE

Diagnosis and Management of Neck and Back Pain

IN PRIMARY CARE

R. Douglas Collins, MD, FACP

Formerly Senior FAA Medical Examiner
Former Associate Professor of Medicine
Medical University of South Carolina
Former Associate Clinical Professor of Medicine
University of Florida School of Medicine
Chatsworth, California

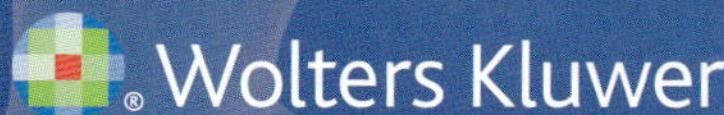

Philadelphia • Baltimore • New York • London
Buenos Aires • Hong Kong • Sydney • Tokyo

Acquisitions Editor: Rebecca Gaertner
Senior Developmental Editor: Kristina Oberle
Marketing Manager: Rachel Mante Leung
Production Project Manager: Kim Cox
Design Coordinator: Stephen Druding
Manufacturing Coordinator: Beth Welsh
Prepress Vendor: SPi Global

9 8 7 6 5 4 3 2 1

Printed in China

Library of Congress Cataloging-in-Publication Data
Names: Collins, R. Douglas, author.
Title: Diagnosis and management of neck and back pain in primary care / R. Douglas Collins.
Description: Philadelphia : Wolters Kluwer, [2017] | Includes bibliographical references and index.
Identifiers: LCCN 2017013156 | ISBN 9781496362742
Subjects: | MESH: Neck Pain—diagnosis | Neck Pain—therapy | Back Pain—diagnosis | Back Pain—therapy | Primary Health Care—methods | Case Reports
Classification: LCC RD771.B217 | NLM WE 708 | DDC 617.5/64—dc23 LC record available at https://lccn.loc.gov/2017013156

LWW.com

RRS1705

To my Lord Jesus Christ, the greatest teacher
and healer of us all.

PREFACE

At least a third of patients seen in primary care practice present with neck or back pain. In fact 90% of Americans will experience back pain at some time in their lives.[1] Unfortunately, too little time is spent on this subject in medical school and residency. Consequently, the majority of primary care clinicians are uncomfortable treating neck and back pain, particularly, low back pain. There is a need for a book that will remedy this deficit and make clinicians more confident in dealing with neck and back pain.

When a patient presents to the primary care provider, he/she needs to be able to determine which patients he/she can treat with confidence and which ones need referrals to an orthopedic or neurological specialist. The clinician needs to know what initial laboratory, x-ray, and other diagnostic procedure to order and when to order MRIs and CT scans and when they are cost-effective.

Unique Features of This Book

1. A reducing diet that is easy to follow and has been successful in thousands of my patients over the last 50 years.
2. Simple back exercises that will strengthen the anterior spinal muscles heretofore never found in print.
3. Techniques for diagnosing and treating scoliosis due to a short leg. This is found in at least 20% of patients with low back pain.
4. The procedure for performing a caudal epidural steroid injection that can safely be performed in the outpatient setting.
5. Illustrations of the examination of a patient with neck, thoracic, and low back pain.
6. Illustrations of the most common causes of neck and back pain.

No other book adequately addresses the needs of a primary care provider. It is an appropriately illustrated, concise review of all the causes of neck and back pain, their diagnosis and management. It will serve as a refresher for primary care clinicians and an easy to read reference to consult in the primary care provider's daily practice. It is the hope of the author that clinicians everywhere will feel more confidence in approaching the patient with neck and back pain after reading this book.

I'd like to thank Carolina Hrejsa and Lik Kwang for their spectacular illustrations and my editors Rebecca Gaertner and Kristina Oberle for turning my manuscript into a beautifully finished textbook! I'm deeply indebted to many others including my wife, Norie, for making this book a reality.

Robert Douglas Collins, MD, FACP

REFERENCE

1. Domino FJ, et al. *The 5 Minute Clinical Consult*. 20th ed. Philadelphia, PA: Wolters Kluwer; 2012.

CONTENTS

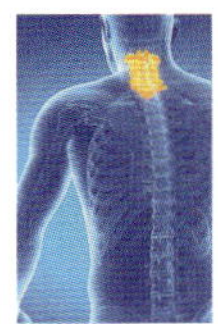

Part I
What Do You Do with the Patient with Neck Pain?

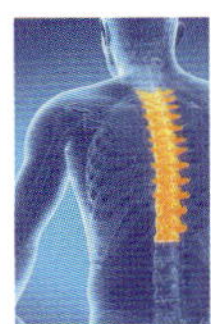

Part II
What Do You Do with the Patient with Thoracic Pain?

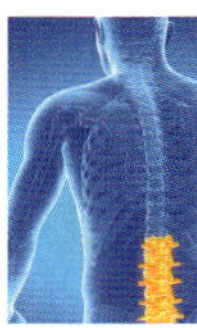

Part III
What Do You Do with the Patient With Low Back Pain?

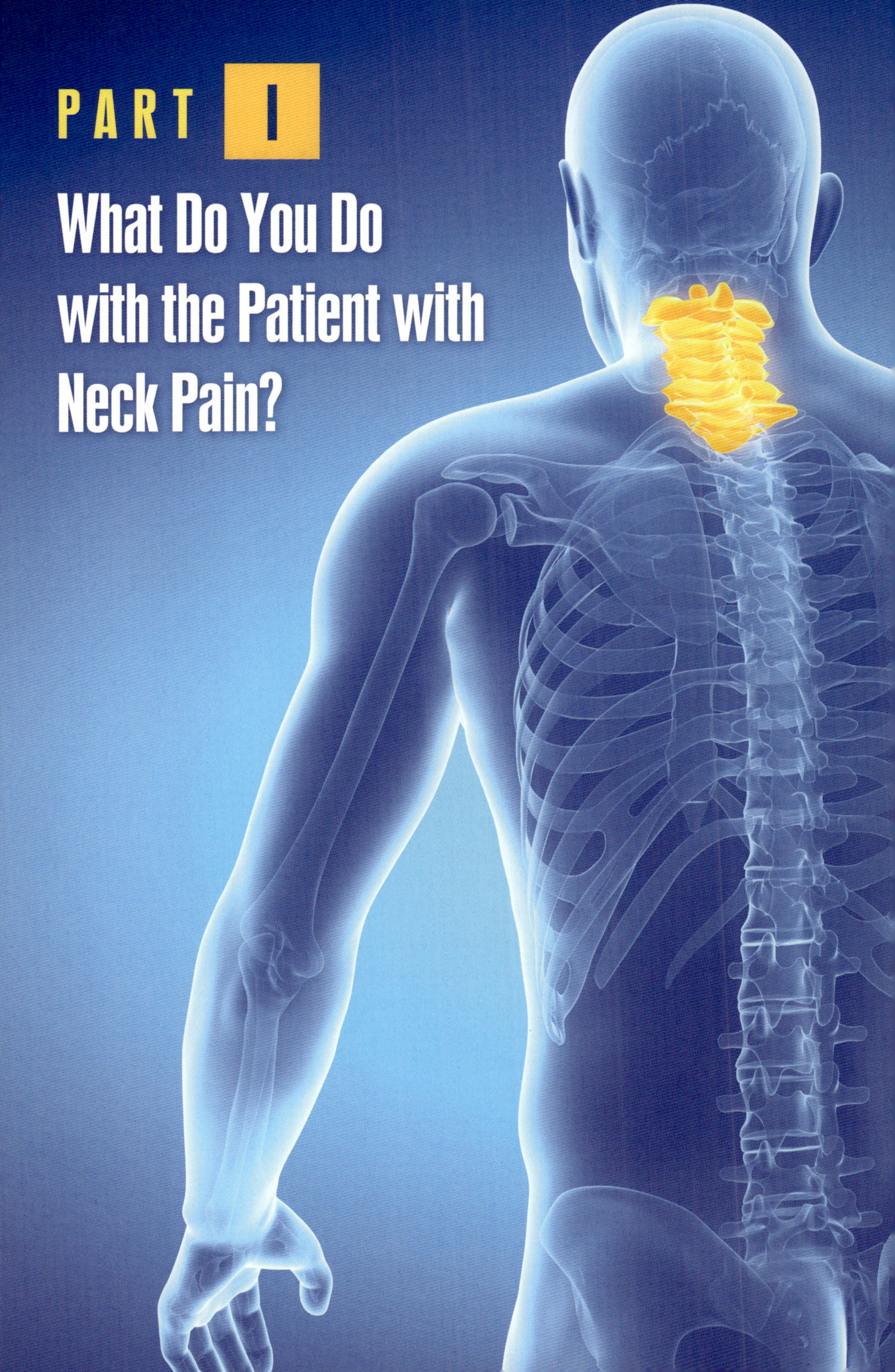

PART I
What Do You Do with the Patient with Neck Pain?

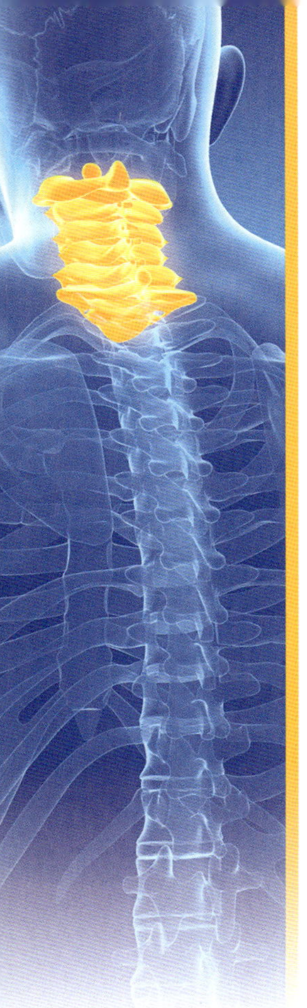

A Taking a History of the Patient with Neck Pain

Rather than interviewing the patient in the traditional way, you should have in mind a list of meaningful questions, and your history taking will be more thorough. One way you can develop this list is by picturing the anatomy of the neck.[1] Considering the skin, you would think of herpes zoster and other diagnostic possibilities (Table 1-1 and Figure 1-1) before you begin.[2] In that way you will ask about

TABLE 1-1

List of the Most Likely Causes of Neck Pain

1. Sprains, contusions
2. Tension headache
3. Migraine
4. Herniated disk
5. Facet syndrome
6. Degenerative spondylosis
7. Spinal stenosis
8. Fractures
9. Osteomyelitis
10. Epidural abscess
11. Meningitis
12. Subarachnoid hemorrhage
13. Thoracic outlet syndrome
14. Primary and metastatic neoplasms
15. Coronary insufficiency
16. Thyroiditis
17. Pancoast tumor
18. Subdiaphragmatic abscess
19. Litigation
20. Conversion or somatization reaction
21. Fibromyositis

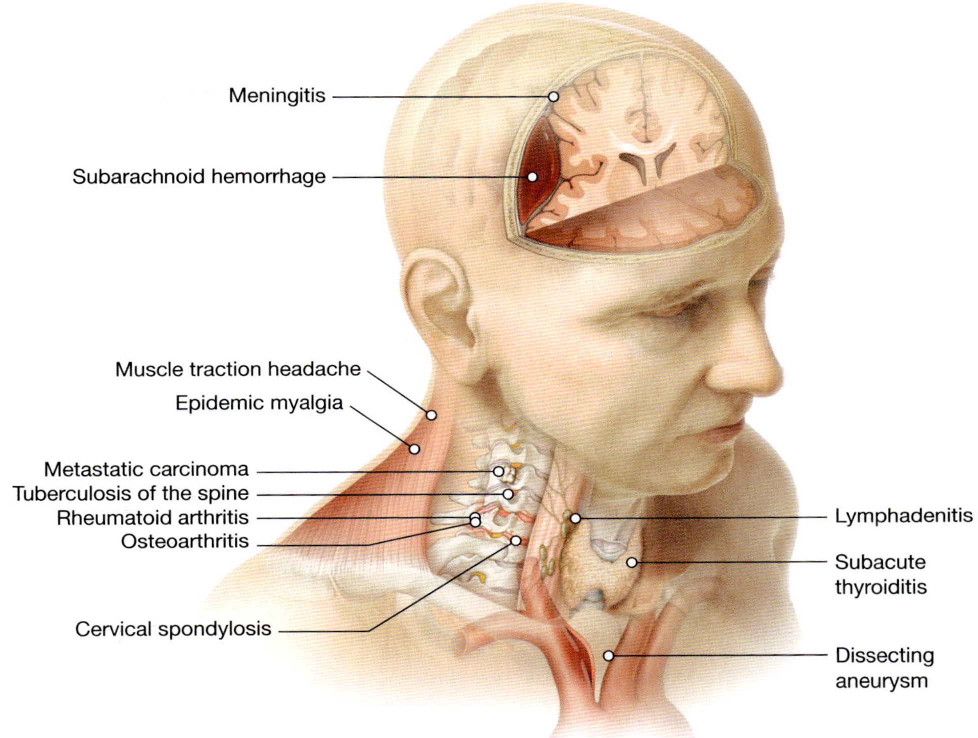

FIGURE 1-1: Illustration of Causes of Neck Pain

cellulitis, for example. Next, you would picture the muscles and recall contusions and sprains, tension headache, or polymyalgia rheumatica. Then the bones, joints, and ligaments would bring to mind cervical spondylosis, rheumatoid arthritis, a herniated disk, etc. Considering the nerves would prompt the recall of brachial plexus neuropathy, a neuroma, thoracic outlet syndrome, Pancoast tumor, or sympathetic dystrophy. Picturing the meninges would help you recall meningitis, subarachnoid hemorrhage, or meningioma. Picturing the blood vessels would allow you to recall migraine and coronary insufficiency. Do not forget the thyroid gland as this would prompt consideration of subacute thyroiditis.

Onset: In developing the chief complaint, we want to know if the neck pain is *acute* or *chronic*. Acute neck pain maybe due to trauma, infection (meningitis, epidural abscess), or a vascular etiology such as a migraine, subarachnoid hemorrhage, or coronary insufficiency, while chronic neck pain is more likely to be due to a space-occupying lesion (tumor or herniated disk) or a degenerative process such as cervical spondylosis. If the pain began after an injury such as a motor vehicle accident (MVA) or heavy lifting, you need the details. Is there radiation of the pain into the extremities? This would suggest a space-occupying lesion such as tumor, abscess, herniated disk, fracture dislocation, or hematoma. One must not forget the possibility of coronary insufficiency, Pancoast tumor, or thoracic outlet syndrome. Aggravation of the pain on coughing or sneezing would suggest radiculopathy from a herniated disk or other space-occupying lesion.

Is the pain constant or intermittent? Constant pain would be indicative of a space-occupying lesion, tension headache, or cervical sprain whereas intermittent pain would suggest migraine, or coronary insufficiency.

What other symptoms are *associated* with the pain? Fever or chills would suggest meningitis or epidural abscess. Nausea, vomiting, or photophobia would suggest migraine. Diaphoresis would suggest coronary insufficiency, while numbness, tingling, or weakness in the upper or lower extremities would suggest a herniated disk or other space-occupying lesion.

Review of Systems: In the review of systems, emphasis should be placed on other neurological symptoms such as weakness, paresthesias, gait disturbances, and symptoms of a neurogenic bladder or erectile dysfunction. Also ask about joint pain (gout and rheumatoid arthritis).

Past History: Certainly, we would want to know about previous accidents, surgeries, hospitalizations, or neoplasms that may be subject to metastasis.

Family History: This may be helpful in differentiating coronary insufficiency and migraine. When all is said and done, our history of neck pain is designed to differentiate between those conditions that can be treated conservatively such as cervical sprain and cervical arthritis (cervical spondylosis, etc.) and more serious conditions such as a herniated disk and other space-occupying lesions that may require surgical intervention; our physical findings will be even more helpful in this regard.

B Examination of the Patient with Neck Pain

Your primary objective in examining a patient with neck pain is to rule out cervical radiculopathy or myelopathy and serious conditions that may cause radiation of pain to the neck such as coronary insufficiency, cholecystitis, and a subdiaphragmatic abscess. In acute cases, you must also consider the possibility of meningitis and subarachnoid hemorrhage. The author can vividly recall a case of acute neck pain that he diagnosed as a subarachnoid hemorrhage simply because he tested for nuchal rigidity. That same patient had been given the diagnosis of migraine when she visited the emergency room 24 hours before.

Your examination begins by examining for a spastic or ataxic gait (Figure 1-2).

Next, perform a Romberg test (Figure 1-3), which will also help rule out myelopathy. Palpate the muscles of the neck for spasm and trigger points (Figure 1-4), which can assist you in diagnosing tension headaches and cervical sprains. Palpate the cervical nerve roots (Figure 1-5) for tenderness, a sign of radiculopathy or brachial plexus neuralgia. Examine the pupils for Horner syndrome, a sign of thoracic outlet syndrome.

Next, test for the range of motion (Figures 1-6 and 1-7), which is normally at 30 degrees of extension, 60 degrees of flexion, and 45 degrees of lateral bending right and left. Limitation of flexion may indicate nuchal rigidity as well as cervical disk herniation, while limitation of extension will be suggestive of cervical spondylosis or ligamentum flavum syndrome. Extension of the neck in the latter condition also causes tingling in the lumbar spine and legs called Lhermitte sign. Limitation of range of motion in all directions is typical of cervical spondylosis or fractures in older patients and fracture in younger patients.

Perform a cervical compression test (Figure 1-8) by applying pressure to the top of the head. If there is radiculopathy, this will cause radiation of

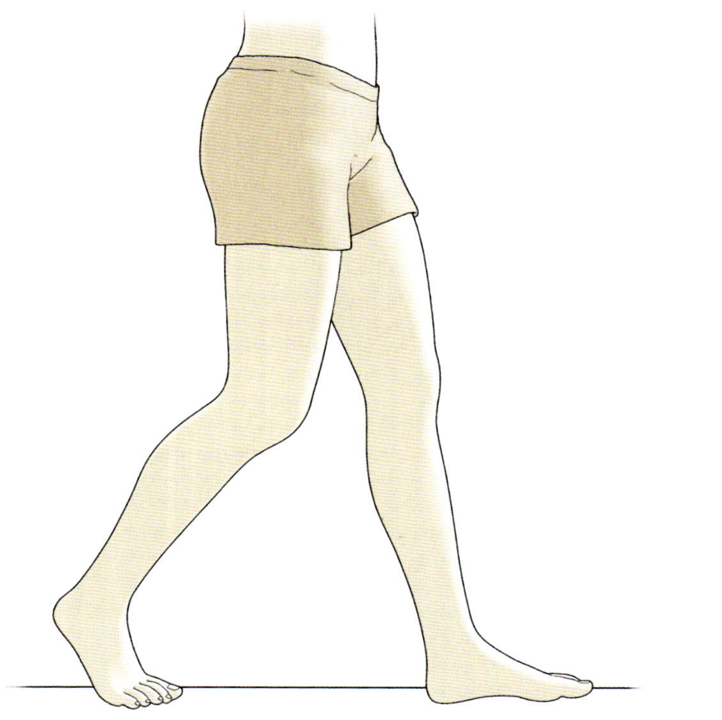

FIGURE 1-2: Gait

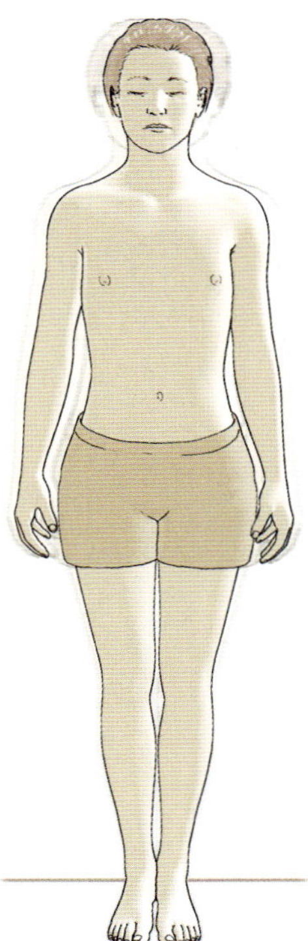

FIGURE 1-3: Romberg

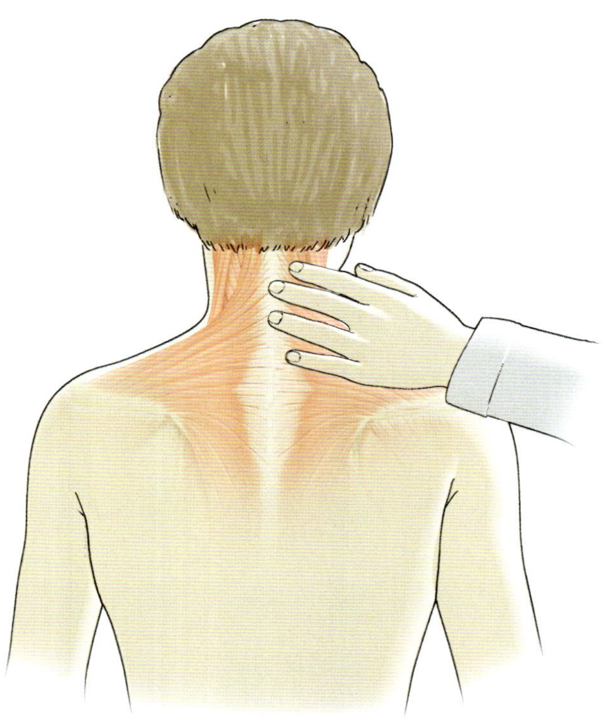

FIGURE 1-4: Palpate for Muscle Spasm and Tenderness

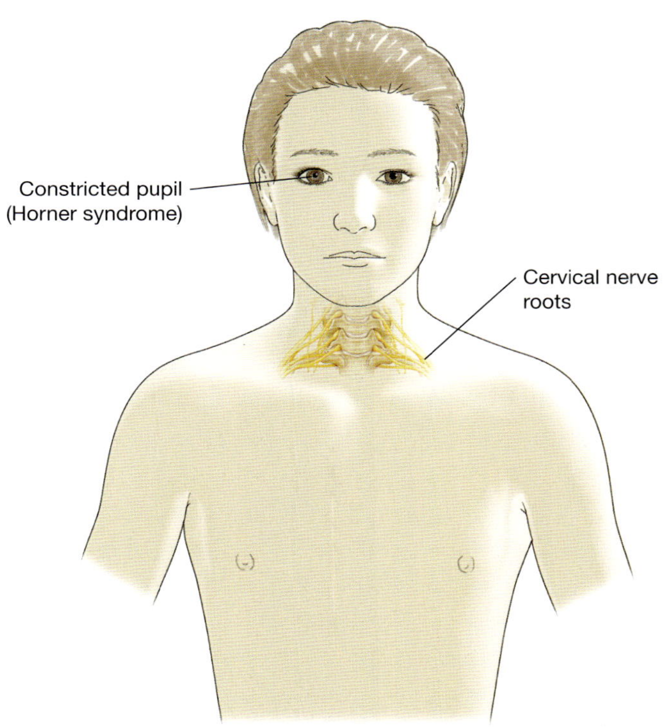

FIGURE 1-5: Palpate Cervical Nerve Root and Look for Unequal Pupils

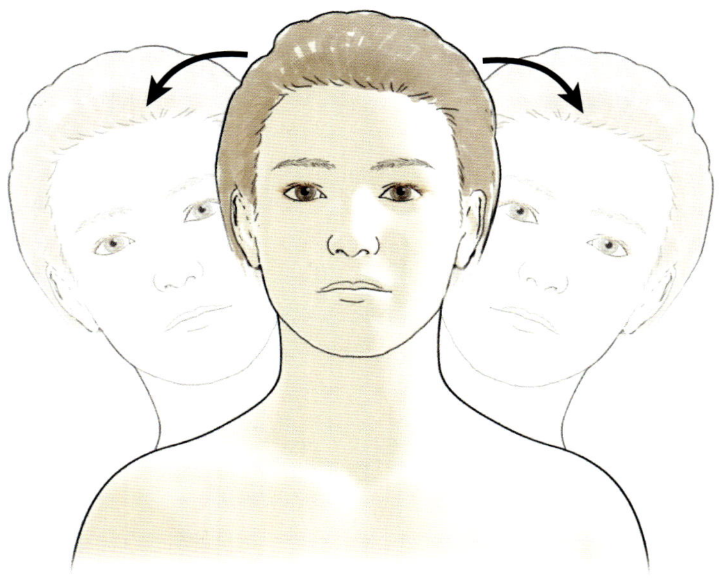

FIGURE 1-6: ROM: Lateral Flexion

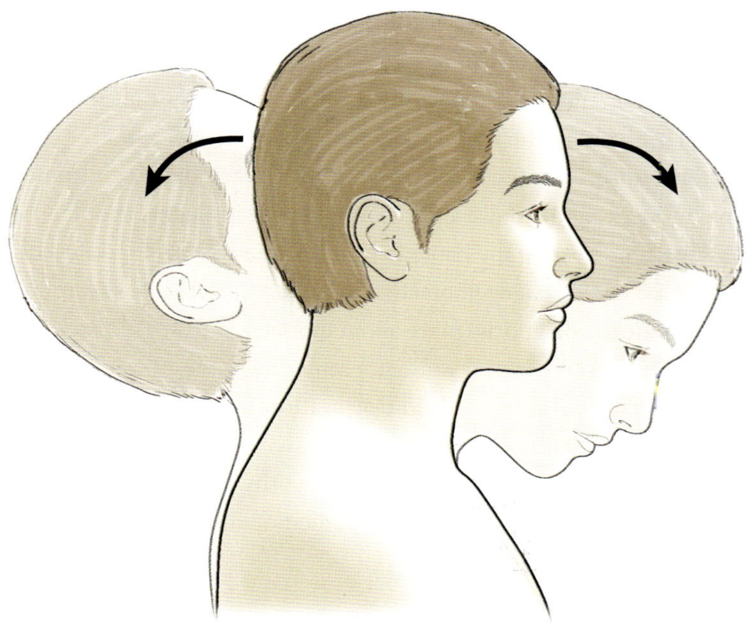

FIGURE 1-7: ROM: Flexion and Extension

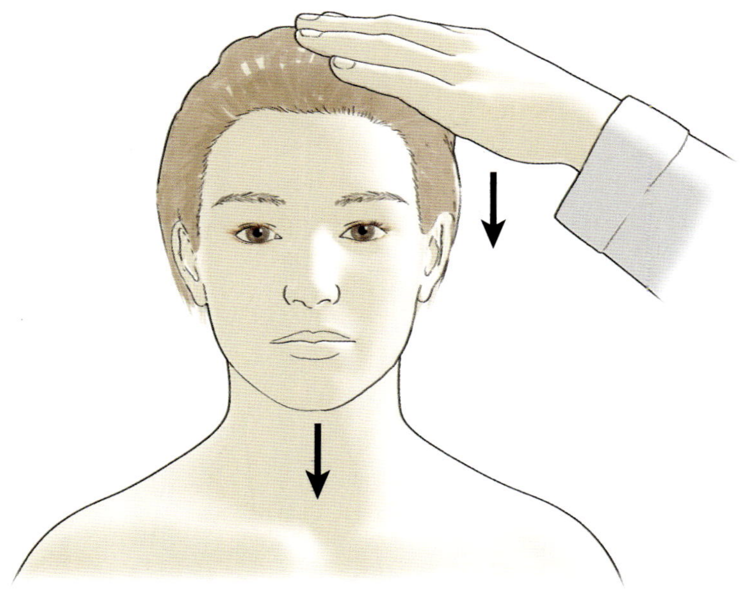

FIGURE 1-8: Cervical Compression Test

pain into one or both upper extremities. The same radiation results when you perform Spurling test (Figure 1-9). This is done by extension, lateral flexion, and rotation of the neck to the right or left and again applying moderate pressure to the top of the head.

Perform Adson tests (Figure 1-10) to rule out thoracic outlet syndrome. This is done by checking the pulse and pressing on the ipsilateral shoulder, while at the same time turning the patient's head to the same or opposite side and having the patient take a deep breath and hold it. If the pulse is diminished, you have made the diagnosis (more about this later in the case histories).

Now, to rule out cervical radiculopathy, check the power (Figures 1-11 and 1-12), reflexes (Figure 1-13), and sensation (Figure 1-14) in the upper extremities. If one or more of these modalities is asymmetrically diminished, you should suspect radiculopathy or neuropathy. For neurologic findings in the most common forms of cervical radiculopathy, see Table 1-2.

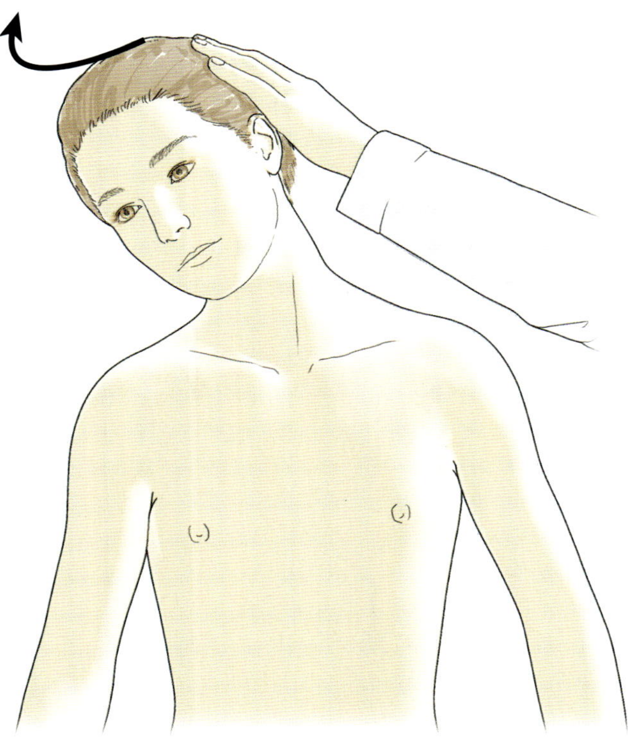

FIGURE 1-9: Spurling Test

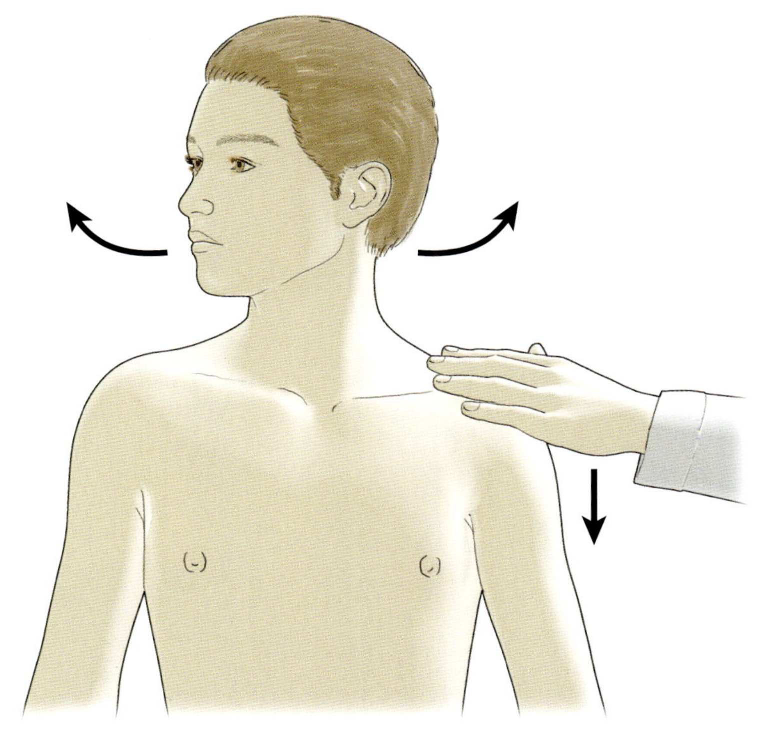

FIGURE 1-10: Adson Tests

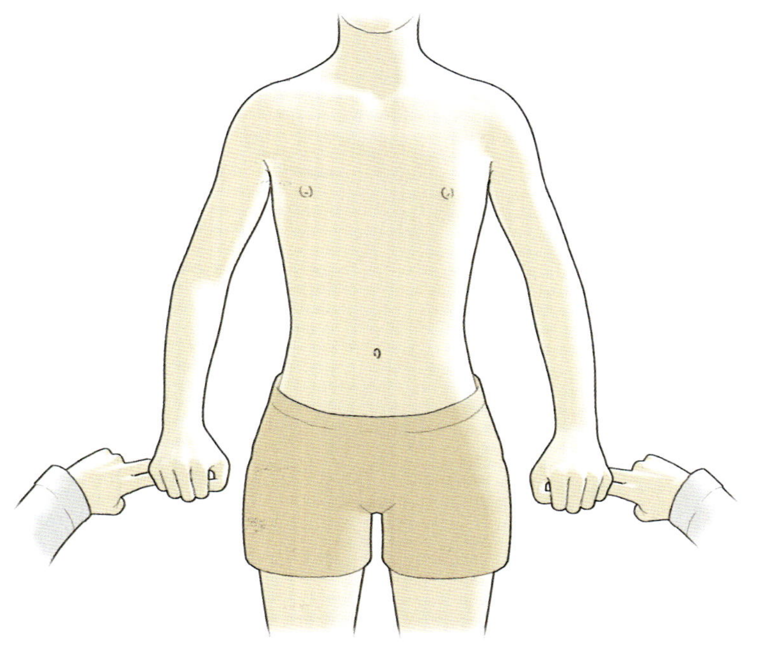

FIGURE 1-11: Power Grip

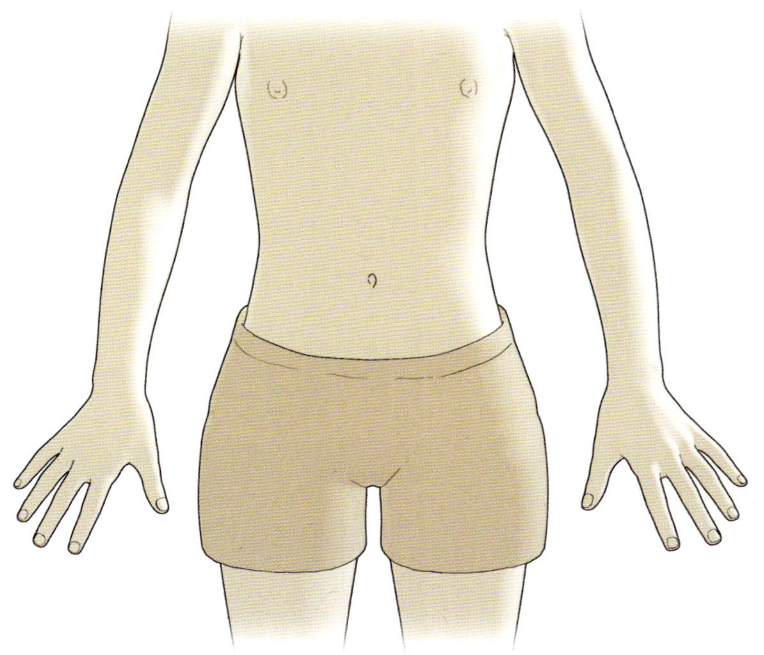

FIGURE 1-12: Power Extension of Fingers and Wrists

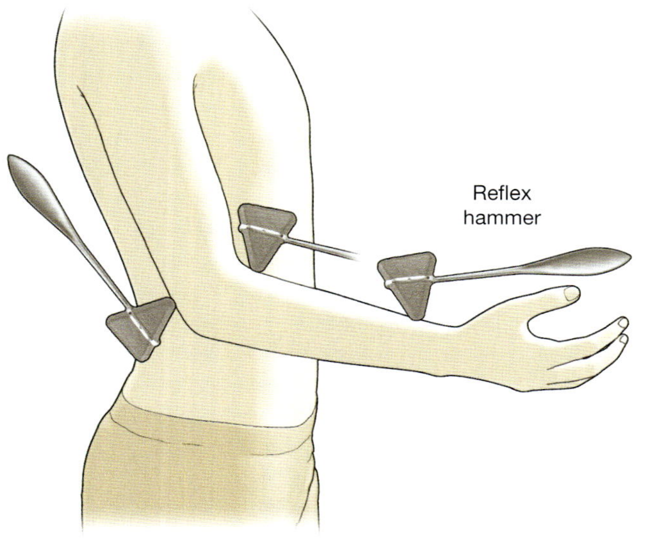

FIGURE 1-13: Reflexes: Upper Extremities

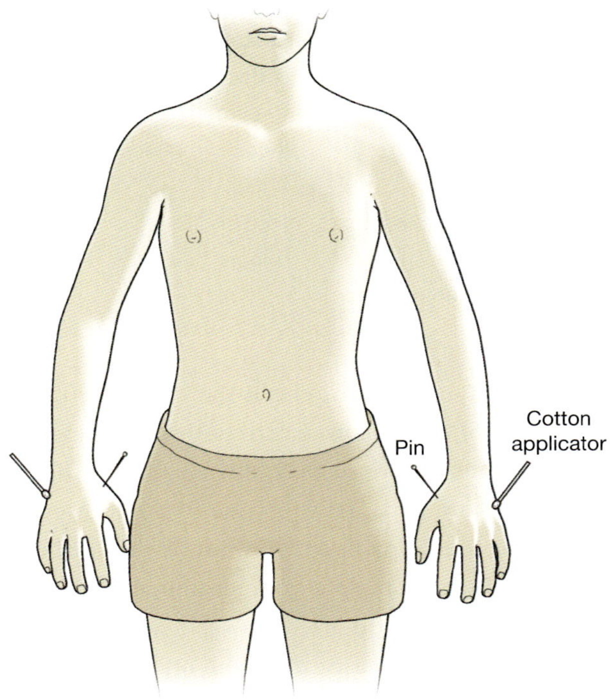

FIGURE 1-14: Sensation: Touch and Pain in Upper Extremities

TABLE 1-2

Neurologic Findings in the Most Common Forms of Cervical Radiculopathy

Nerve Root Involved	Weakness	Loss of Sensation	Loss of Reflexes
C5	Deltoid and biceps	Lateral shoulder and arm	Biceps
C6	Wrist extension, biceps and triceps	Thumb and radial surface of the forearm	Brachioradialis
C7	Triceps and wrist flexion	Index and middle finger	Triceps
C8	Flexion of the fingers, abduction and abduction of fingers	Ring and little fingers	None

Next, to rule out myelopathy, check the reflexes (Figure 1-15) and sensation (Figure 1-16) in the lower extremities. Be sure to check for a Babinski sign. You should suspect myelopathy if the Babinski is positive, the reflexes are hyperactive in one or both lower extremities, or the sensation to touch, pain, or vibration is diminished in one or both lower extremities. Complete your examination by auscultation of the heart, lungs, and carotid arteries (Figure 1-17) to help rule out a myocardial infarct, pleurisy, pericarditis, and other conditions that may refer pain to the neck. There will be times when you suspect intracranial pathology and you need to examine the cranial nerves or do a complete neurologic examination. The steps to take in this case are demonstrated in *Appendix A*.

C Diagnosis of the Patient with Neck Pain

Once you have completed your history and physical examination, you are left with four possible scenarios, which will determine how you proceed with your workup and treatment:

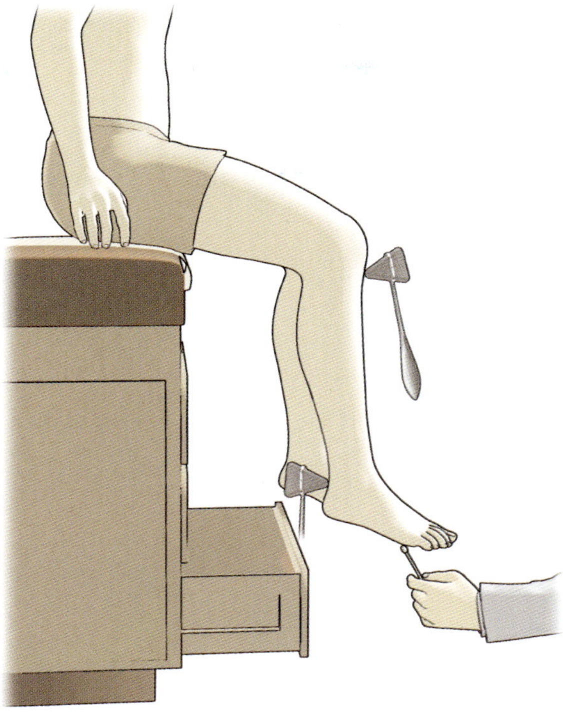

FIGURE 1-15: Reflexes: Lower Extremities

1. **Neck pain with no radiation to the upper extremities, no history of trauma, and no objective neurologic findings.** In these cases, some authorities advise proceeding to a course of conservative treatment without any diagnostic workup at all as these cases are most likely cervical sprains, cervical spondylosis, or other forms of arthritis. However, the author advises a workup including a CBC, sedimentation rate, comprehensive metabolic panel, and plain films of the cervical spine. The sedimentation rate is especially useful to exclude polymyalgia rheumatica and an infectious disease process.
2. **Neck pain without radiation to the upper extremities or positive neurologic findings, but with a history of trauma.** The diagnosis in these cases is most likely a cervical sprain, which can be handled conservatively, but an x-ray to rule out fracture or other subtle pathology is justified. In cases of severe injury or pain, a CT scan should be done to be sure there is no fracture.

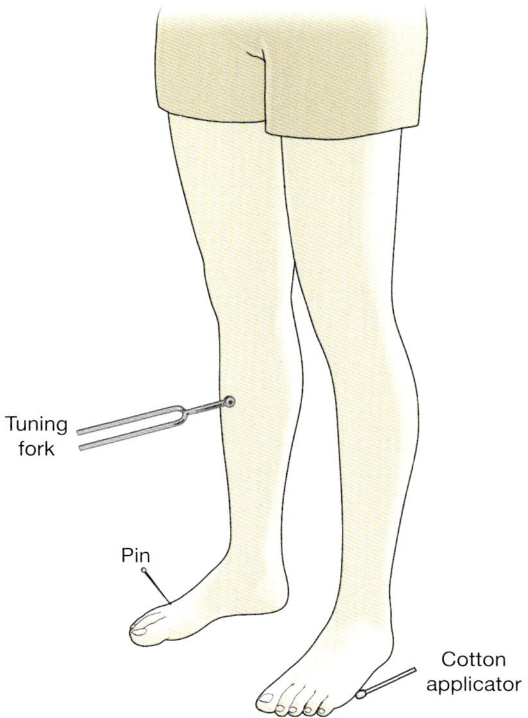

FIGURE 1-16: Sensation: Touch and Pain, Vibration—Lower Extremities

3. **Neck pain with radiation of pain to one or both upper extremities, mild objective signs of radiculopathy with or without a history of trauma, but no evidence of myelopathy.** The diagnosis of these cases includes neoplasm, herniated disk, cervical spondylosis, fracture, and brachial plexus neuropathy. An x-ray of the cervical spine, CBC, sedimentation rate, arthritis panel, and chemistry panel are done before launching on a course of conservative treatment.
4. **Neck pain with clear neurologic signs of radiculopathy or myelopathy and significant weakness or atrophy in the upper or lower extremities.** These patients most likely have a fracture or space-occupying lesion of the spinal cord such as herniated disk or tumor but of course could have advanced cervical spondylosis with spinal

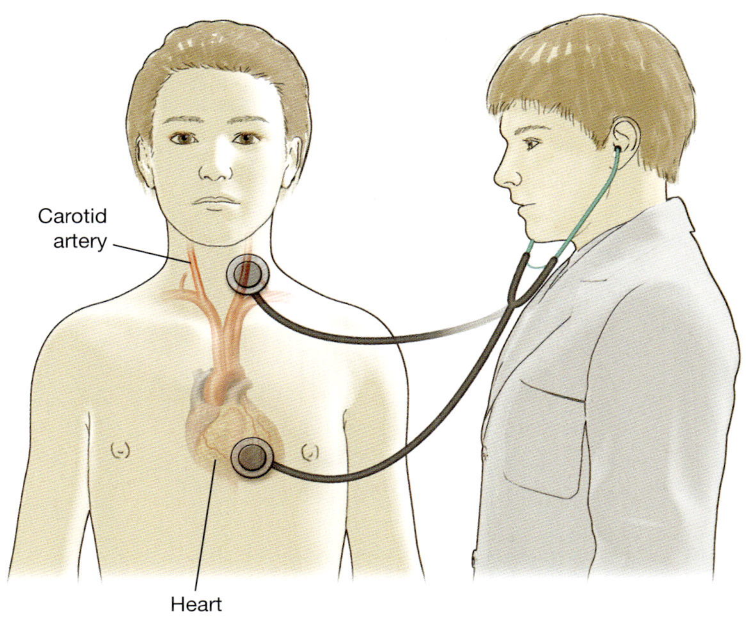

FIGURE 1-17: Auscultation of Heart, Chest, and Carotids

stenosis and require immediate referral to a neurosurgeon. There is no reason to order expensive diagnostic studies such as an MRI or CT scan when a referral will be made anyway.

D Conservative Management of the Patient with Neck Pain

Table 1-3 lists all the possible forms of conservative therapy.

Acute Neck Pain: In cases of acute neck pain, the treatment of choice is nonnarcotic analgesics such as acetaminophen and NSAIDs such as ibuprofen, 600 to 800 mg T.I.D. or naproxen 250 to 500 mg B.I.D.[3] These should be taken with meals or a large glass of water to avoid an ulcer. Narcotics may be given for a short period, but it is recommended that these be avoided at all costs because of the risk of addiction. Alternatively,

TABLE 1-3

Conservative Management of Neck Pain

1. Analgesic
2. Nonsteroidal anti-inflammatory drugs
3. Muscle relaxants
4. Corticosteroids
5. Reducing diets
6. Cervical collar
7. Cervical traction
8. Physiotherapy—Refer to a physiotherapist or physiatrist for a treatment plan
9. Exercises
10. Trigger point injections
11. Facet injections
12. Nerve root injections
13. Stellate ganglion blocks
14. Epidural injections
15. Prayer
16. Antidepressants and anticonvulsants

if narcotics are required, hospitalize the patient. Muscle relaxants such as cyclobenzaprine (Flexeril) 10 mg T.I.D. and metaxalone (Skelaxin) 800 mg T.I.D. may be prescribed, but their effectiveness is questionable.[4] The author has found carisoprodol (Soma) more effective, but there is a risk of dependency with this drug. Benzodiazepines are often effective, but again dependency is a real possibility.

When NSAIDs are not effective, a short course of oral corticosteroids may be prescribed. Alternate-day steroids such as prednisone 5 to 20 mg Q.O.D. have been successful in the author's experience especially when combined with NSAIDs.[5] The usual side effects from steroids (diabetes, hypertension, ulcers, osteoporosis, and adrenal insufficiency) are rare with this regimen.[6]

A soft cervical collar latched in front is recommended and is especially helpful when worn at night. This will prevent the patient from getting the neck in a stressful position during sleep.

Trigger point injections, occipital nerve blocks, and cervical nerve root injections with 1% to 2% lidocaine with or without corticosteroids (10 to 40 mg of triamcinolone acetonide) may be therapeutic as well as diagnostic. If the provider is inexperienced with these procedures, referral to an anesthesiologist or neurological specialist may be necessary to accomplish these. Physiotherapy has its advocates but is expensive and may lead to dependency or run up the cost of litigation.

Chronic Neck Pain: Here again, analgesics, NSAIDs, muscle relaxants, and short courses of low-dose corticosteroids may be prescribed. A soft cervical collar to be worn at night may also be helpful. Be sure to latch in front. To relieve the pressure on the cervical spine, a reducing diet should be prescribed in the obese patient. Table 1-4 describes the fruit and vegetable diet favored by the author. Trigger point, nerve root, and facet injections can be very effective. Epidural injections may also be tried but are best done by a specialist trained in this procedure. Cervical traction may be useful if there is radiculopathy. There is an over-the-counter

TABLE 1-4

The Fruit and Vegetable Diet[7]

1. For 6 days a week, limit your food to fresh fruits or low-calorie canned fruit (without sugar added), vegetables, and nuts. The amount you consume is not limited with the exception of potatoes and rice. Peanut butter on crackers or whole wheat bread is acceptable and suppresses the appetite.
2. Eliminate all dairy products, beef, chicken, and pork.
3. Fish is acceptable, but you will not lose weight as fast.
4. On the 7th day, you may eat anything you want, but don't overdo it. This follows the Bible precedent of "6 days shalt thou labor and do all the work and on the 7th day you rest."
5. On average, you can lose 2–3 lbs a week on this diet, but realize there will be some weeks when you don't lose any. Weight loss always comes in a stair-step fashion.

Adapted from Collins RD. *What Every Patient Should Know about His/Her Health, and His/Her Doctor.* New York: Exposition Press; 1973.

apparatus that can be obtained at Home Medical Supply stores or pharmacies. The patient begins with 10 lbs for one half hour twice a day and gradually works up to 15 lbs for 1 hour twice or three times a day. Hospitalization with a traction setup in the recumbent position is even better, but it is debatable whether an insurance company will pay for this. All patients with neck and back pain will have a better chance of recovery with proper nutrition and vitamins particularly vitamin D_3 1,000 to 2,000 units a day.

Physiotherapy for chronic neck pain is acceptable if you will let a physiatrist or the physiotherapist tailor the therapy to the individual's needs. In my opinion, they are best qualified in this regard.

Passive and active exercises as depicted in Table 1-5 provide excellent results in many cases. These are especially successful in cases of chronic sprains and cervical spondylosis.

TABLE 1-5

Exercises for the Patient with Neck Pain

Purpose: to increase the comfortable range of motion of your neck.

1. Passive Exercise (Isotonic):
   a. Slowly bend your neck laterally back and forth to the right and left for 2 min.
   b. Next slowly extend and flex your neck back and forth for 2 min.
   c. Finally rotate your neck slowly to the right and left for 2 min.
   d. Do not go beyond a comfortable point with each of these exercises.
   e. Repeat these exercises three times a day.
2. Exercises against resistance (isometric). (Only with your doctor's permission.)
   a. Perform the first two of the above exercises against the resistance from your hand, applying force to each side of your head (for the lateral bending) and then to the back and front of your head (for the extension and flexion exercise).
   b. Again, this is done for 2 min for each exercise three times a day.
   c. This will increase the stability of the vertebrae.

If the above measures are ineffective, the author has found prayer to achieve miraculous results in some cases. However, it is important to ask the patient's permission first.

Finally, antidepressants and anticonvulsants such as gabapentin may be tried for neuropathic pain, but the success is variable.[8] Duloxetine 40 to 60 mg B.I.D. has recently been approved by the FDA for back pain and is certainly worth trying as long as one is aware of the potential side effects. When all else fails, a referral to a specialist in pain management, psychiatrist, or neurosurgeon may be worthwhile if for no other reason than to impress upon the patient that everything possible is being done. An algorithm of the management of neck pain is depicted in Figure 1-18.

The various options for surgical intervention are listed in Table 1-6.

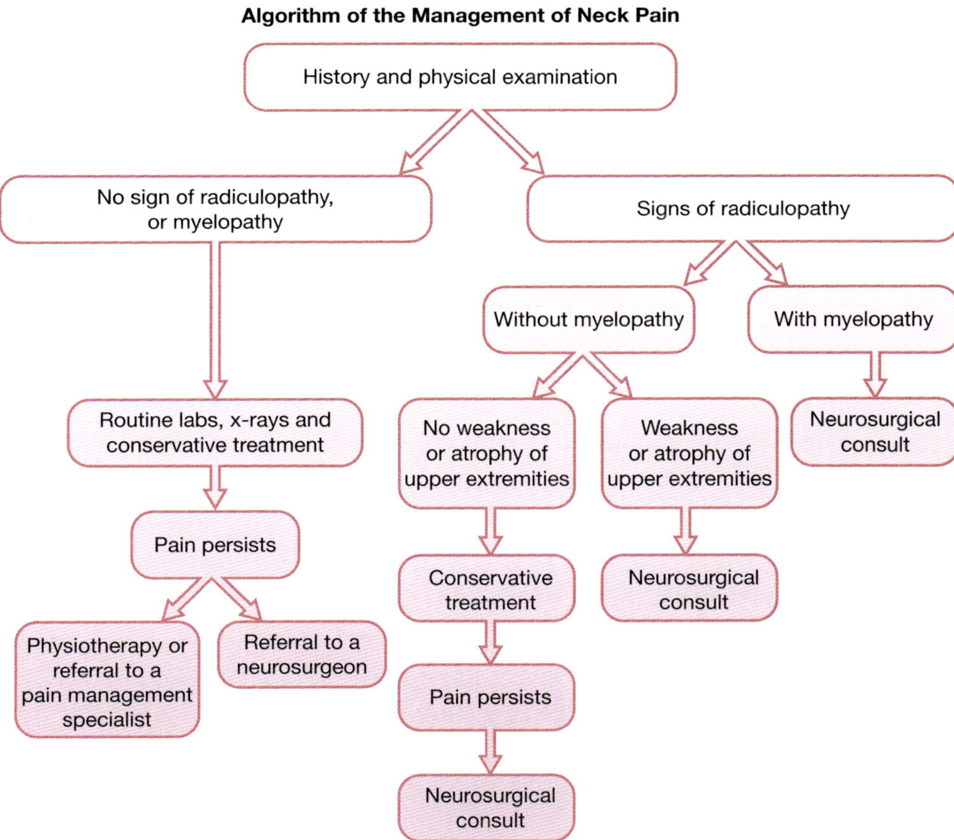

FIGURE 1-18: Management of Neck Pain Algorithm

TABLE 1-6

Surgical Management of Neck Pain

1. Anterior cervical discectomy and fusion
2. Anterior foraminotomy
3. Anterior cervical discectomy and artificial disk replacement
4. Posterior cervical foraminotomy
5. Laminectomy (for spinal cord tumors)

E Illustrated Cases of Neck Pain

Normal Anatomy of the Cervical Spine (Figure 1-19)

Lateral Herniated Cervical Disk (Figure 1-20)

A 36-year-old white male complained of pain in his neck radiating into his right arm and hand particularly the right thumb. The pain was increased on coughing. There was also numbness and tingling of the right arm and thumb. History revealed that he was in an auto accident 2 weeks ago and the pain began immediately after that. He had gone to the ER, had x-rays, and was fitted with a soft cervical collar.

Physical examination revealed increase of the pain on cervical spine compression and Spurling tests. There was tenderness of the C6 nerve root on the right, diminished right biceps reflex, and loss of sensation to touch and pain in the right C6 dermatome. An MRI of the cervical spine revealed a herniated disk at C5-C6 with compression of the C6 nerve root.

Treatment with cervical traction, muscle relaxants, and nonsteroidal anti-inflammatory drugs was successful, and surgery was avoided.

Differential Diagnosis

1. Cervical sprain
2. Cervical spondylosis
3. Thoracic outlet syndrome
4. Compression fracture of the cervical spine.

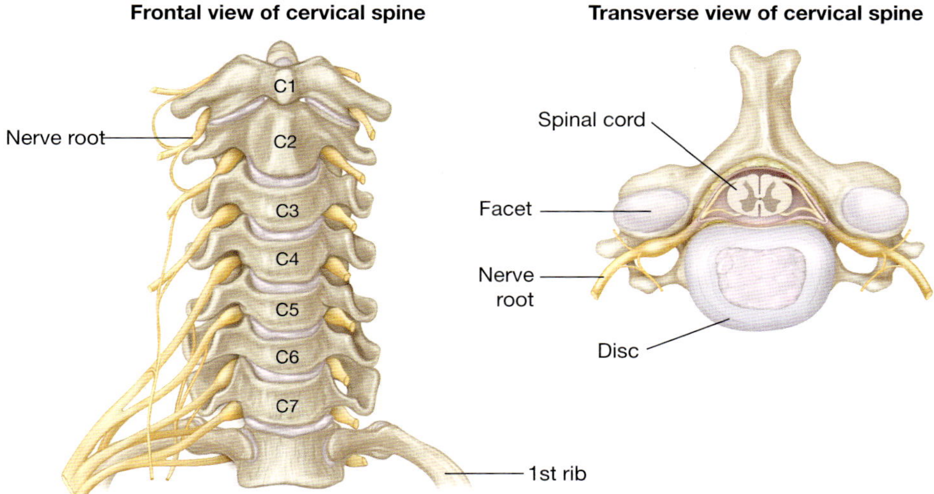

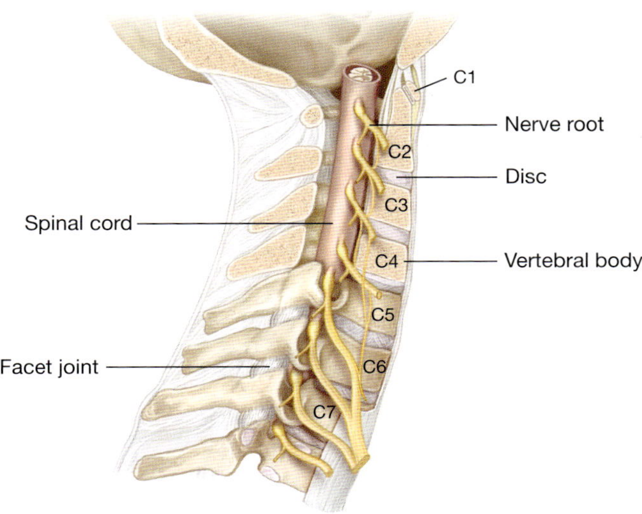

FIGURE 1-19: Normal Anatomy of the Cervical Spine

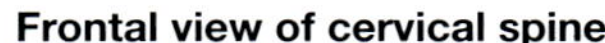

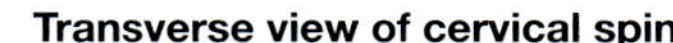

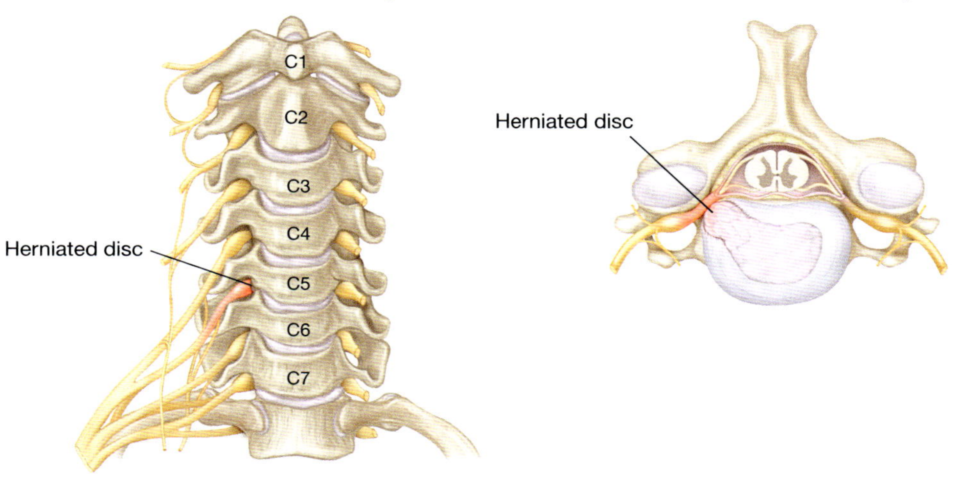

Sagittal view of cervical spine

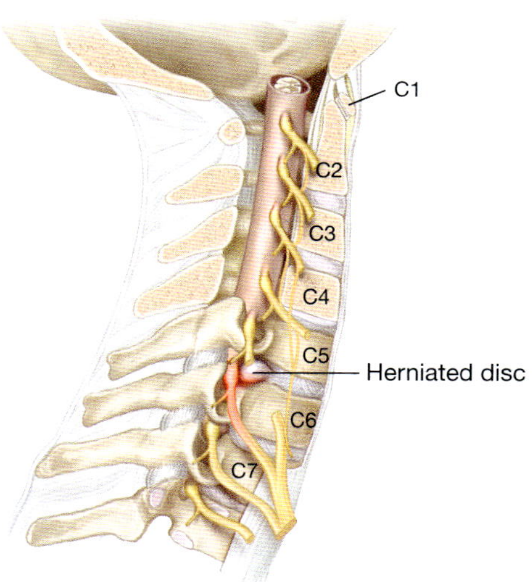

FIGURE 1-20: Lateral Herniated Cervical Disk

Discussion: Although not common, this lesion is occasionally the result of a flexion–extension injury (whiplash).

Conservative treatment is often successful, but a laminectomy or anterior body fusion may be necessary.

Central Herniated Cervical Disk (Figure 1-21)

A 45-year-old nurse complained of moderate to severe neck pain and numbness and tingling in both lower extremities after turning a patient in bed. She showed up 2 weeks later for evaluation.

Physical examination revealed increase of the neck pain on cervical compression and radiation of the pain into her left upper extremity. In addition, there was a spastic gait, and weakness, increased deep tendon reflexes, and moderate loss of vibratory sense in both lower extremities. She denied chills or fever or previous neurologic disease.

Plain films of the cervical spine revealed narrowing of the C5-C6 interspace, and an MRI of the cervical spine showed a cervical disk herniation at C5-C6.

Treatment with immediate laminectomy was successful.

Differential Diagnosis

1. Fracture of the cervical spine
2. Primary or metastatic neoplasm
3. Cervical spondylosis
4. Anterior spinal artery occlusion
5. Parasagittal meningioma
6. Epidural abscess
7. Multiple sclerosis

Discussion: The sudden onset of pain and numbness and tingling in the lower extremities following an injury make a neoplasm or multiple sclerosis unlikely. Immediate referral to a neurosurgeon is imperative.

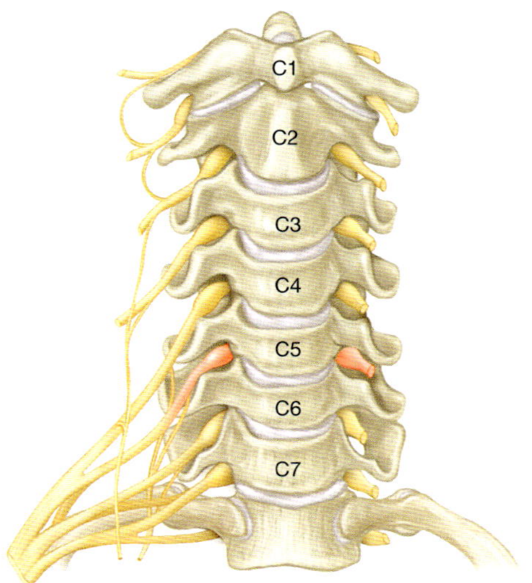

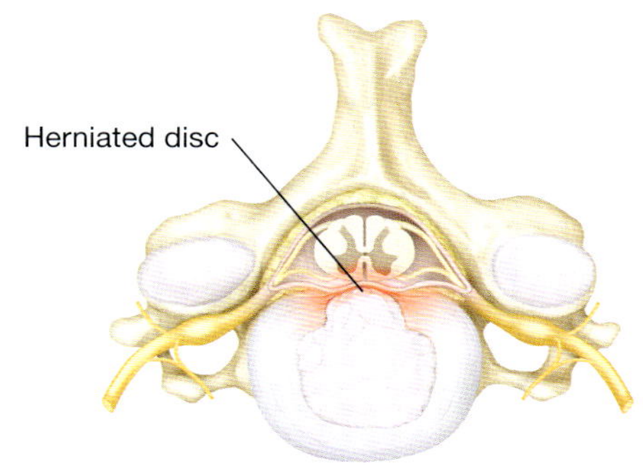

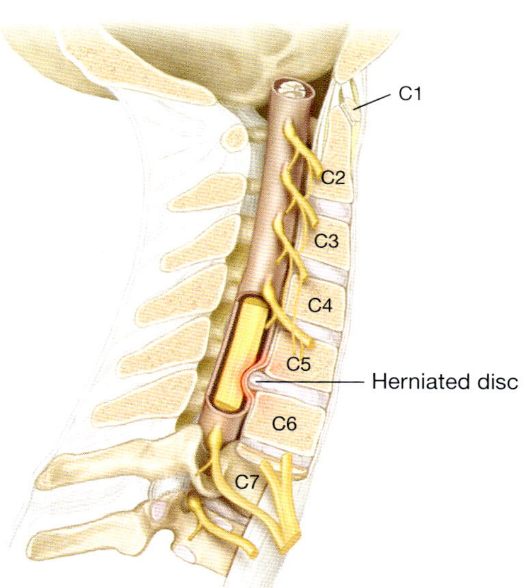

FIGURE 1-21: Central Herniated Cervical Disk

Cervical Facet Syndrome (Figure 1-22)

A 62-year-old black auto mechanic complained of recurrent pain in the right side of his neck with occasional pain radiating down his right arm.

Neurologic examination failed to show any objective findings other than tenderness of the right C5-C6 facet joint, reproduction of the pain on extension of his neck, and tenderness of the right C6 nerve root. An injection of 3 cc of 2% lidocaine around his right C5-C6 facet was both diagnostic and therapeutic. Nevertheless, he was treated with naproxen 500 mg B.I.D. and a cervical collar to wear at night. Follow-up visit 4 weeks later revealed his recovery to be sustained.

Differential Diagnosis

1. Cervical sprain
2. Cervical spondylosis
3. Early neoplasm of the cervical spine
4. Coronary insufficiency
5. Thoracic outlet syndrome
6. Polymyalgia rheumatica

Discussion: Without objective neurologic findings and a history of trauma, there is no need for laboratory, x-ray examinations, or special diagnostic procedures when the patient responds to treatment as this patient did.

Neoplasm of the Cervical Spine (Figure 1-23)

A 67-year-old Hispanic male had been treated for chronic neck pain for 18 months by his local chiropractor. When he began developing weakness, numbness and tingling in his lower extremities, and difficulty walking, he was referred for neurologic evaluation.

Neurologic examination revealed mild weakness in his right upper extremity, loss of his triceps reflex, and hyperactive reflexes in his lower extremities with bilateral Babinski signs. An MRI of the cervical spine revealed a meningioma at the C7 level, and he underwent a cervical laminectomy for removal.

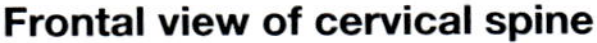

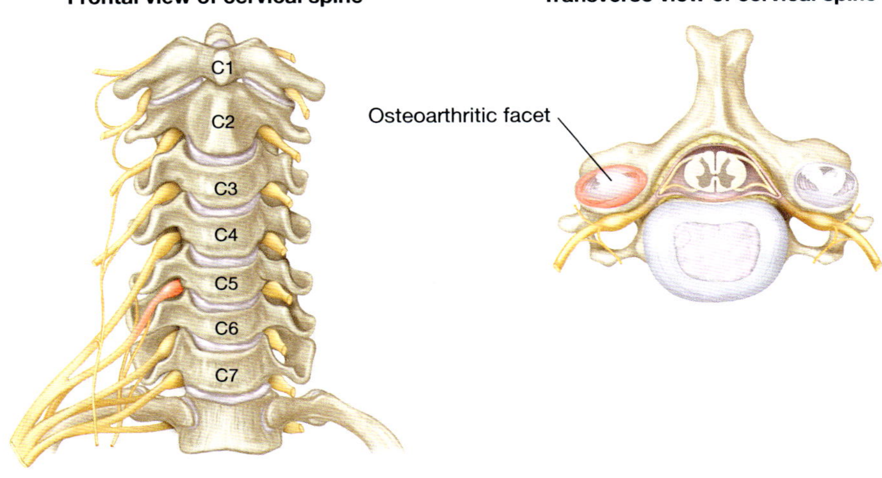

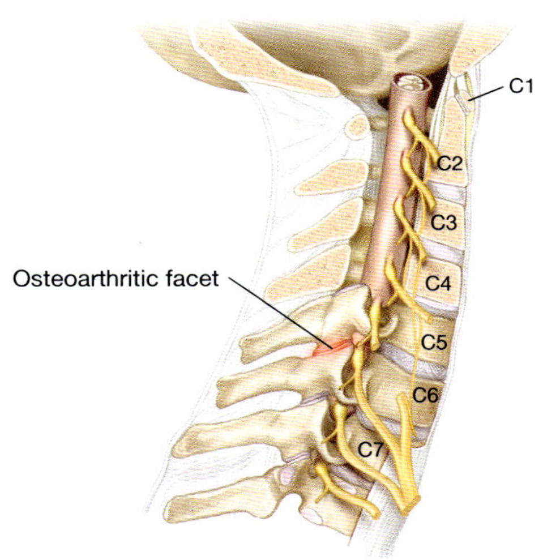

FIGURE 1-22: Cervical Facet Syndrome

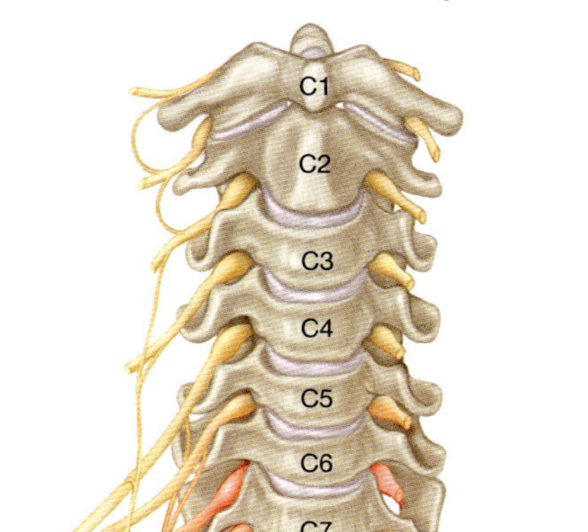

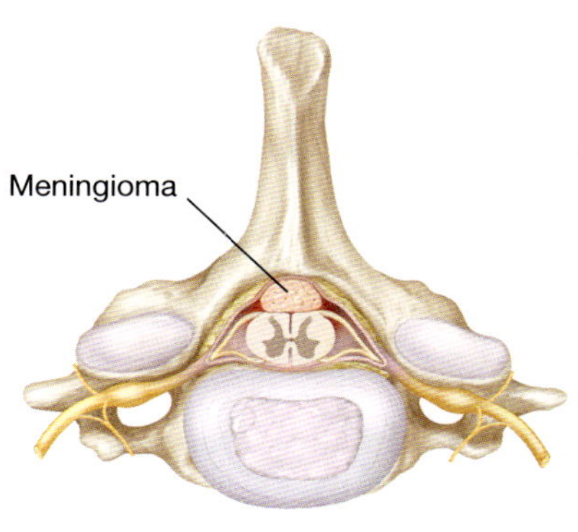

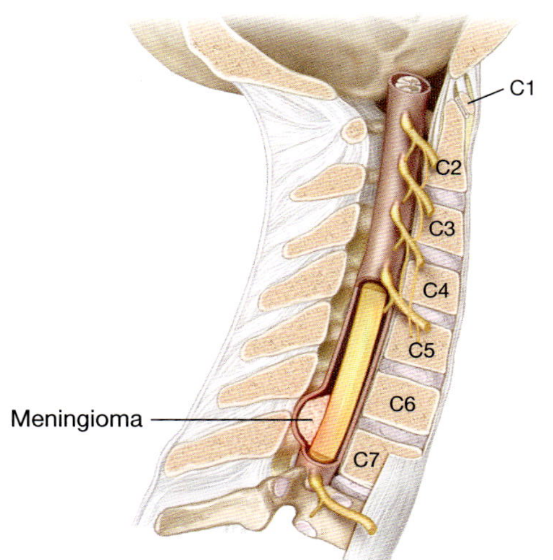

FIGURE 1-23: Neoplasm of the Cervical Spine

Differential Diagnosis

1. Herniated cervical disk
2. Cervical spondylosis
3. Metastatic neoplasm
4. Anterior spinal artery occlusion
5. Tuberculosis of the spinal column

Discussion: Deterioration of a patient on chiropractic treatment or conservative treatment by a primary care provider is scary, but there is usually a logical explanation, so there is no need to panic until adequate studies are completed.

Thoracic Outlet Syndrome (Figure 1-24)

A 24-year-old medical student complained of intermittent pain, numbness, and tingling in his left arm for several years. He finally came for neurologic evaluation because he thought he had multiple sclerosis. His past history revealed he had optic neuritis of his left eye at age 17 but made a full recovery after a tonsillectomy.

Neurologic examination revealed a diminished radial pulse in his left arm on turning his head to the right and taking a deep breath (Adson test for scalenus anticus syndrome). The rest of his neurologic examination was unremarkable. X-rays of his cervical spine were normal. There was no cervical rib.

Treatment: After 2 months of isometric trapezius exercises (shoulder shrugs), he became asymptomatic.

Differential Diagnosis

1. Multiple sclerosis
2. TIA
3. Coronary insufficiency
4. Herniated cervical disk
5. Spinal cord neoplasm
6. Carpal tunnel syndrome

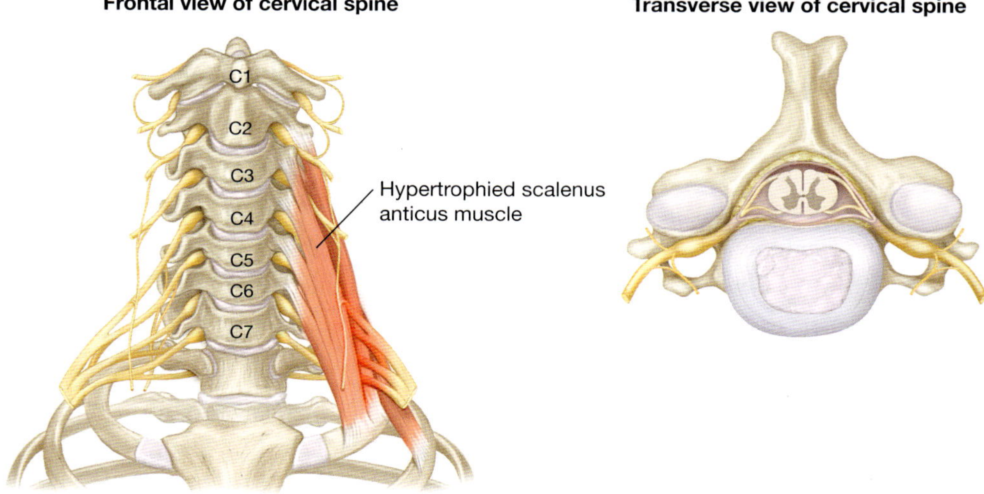

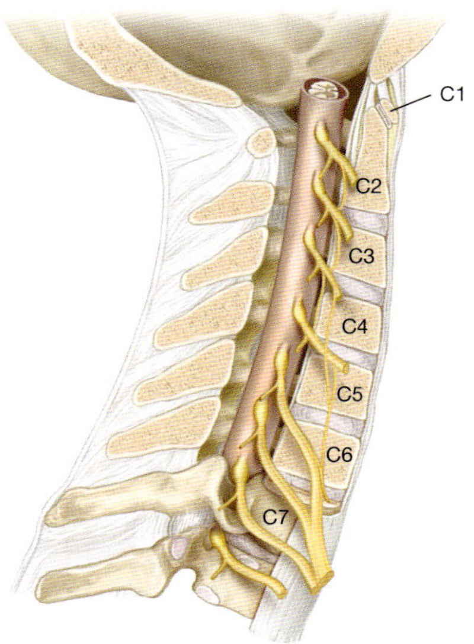

FIGURE 1-24: Thoracic Outlet Syndrome

7. Ulnar entrapment
8. Sympathetic dystrophy
9. Subacromial bursitis
10. Pancoast tumor

Discussion: This is a good example of a case where an MRI of the cervical spine would have been an unnecessary expense. It's always best to refer a patient to a neurologist or neurosurgeon before under taking expensive diagnostic tests.

Cervical Spondylosis (Figure 1-25)

A 59-year-old Hispanic female was referred for neurologic evaluation because of neck and right arm pain for several months. There was no history of injury.

Physical examination revealed limited range of motion of the cervical spine to 10 degrees extension and 25 degrees lateral bending bilaterally. There was spasm of the trapezius and splenius capitis muscles bilaterally and a positive cervical compression test. Sensation to touch and pain was diminished in the right C7 dermatome, but otherwise, the neurologic examination was unremarkable. X-rays of the cervical spine revealed osteoarthritic changes at C5-C6 and C6-C7, and an MRI showed encroachment of the C6-C7 foramina on the right. Treatment with cervical traction, NSAIDs, and muscle relaxants was successful in alleviating her pain.

Differential Diagnosis

1. Cervical sprain
2. Herniated cervical disk
3. Compression fracture
4. Metastatic carcinoma
5. Spinal cord tumor
6. Tuberculosis of the cervical spine

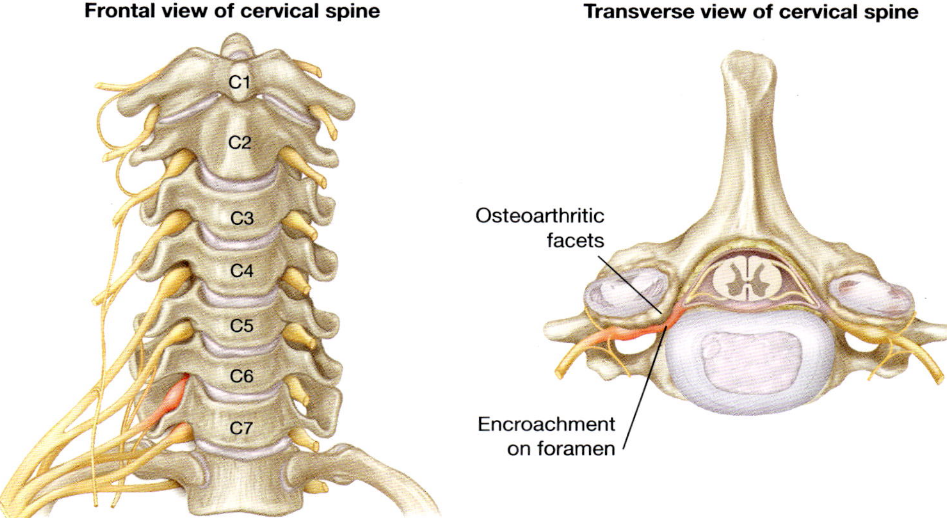

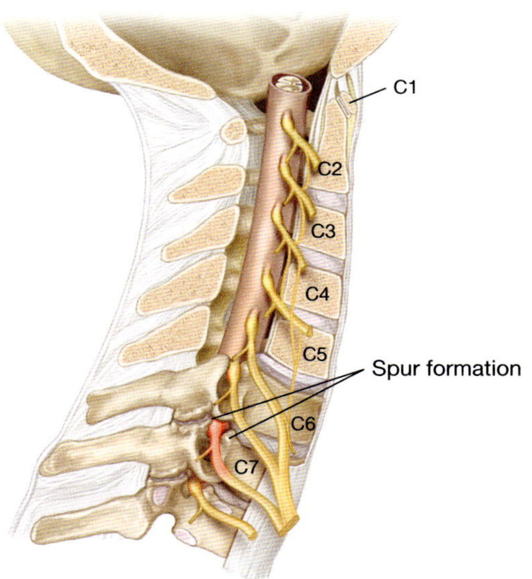

FIGURE 1-25: Cervical Spondylosis

Discussion: Plain films are usually positive in these cases, but an MRI is more definitive. However, it is not cost-effective to order an MRI unless surgery is contemplated. These patients often improve on conservative therapy, but surgery is ultimately necessary in many cases.

REFERENCES

1. Collins RD. *Differential Diagnosis in Primary Care*. Philadelphia, PA: Wolters Kluwer/Lippincott Williams & Wilkins; 2012.
2. Collins RD. *Atlas of Neurologic Diagnosis and Treatment*. Philadelphia, PA: Lippincott Williams & Wilkins; 2005:1.
3. Bope ET, Kellerman RD. *Conn's Current Therapy*. Philadelphia, PA: Elsevier Saunders; 2012.
4. Van Tulder MW, Touray T, Furlan AD, et al. Muscle relaxants for non-specific low back pain. *Cochrane Database of Sys Rev*. 2006;(3):CD004252.
5. Katzung BG, et al. *Basic and Clinical Pharmacology*. 12th ed. New York: McGraw Hill; 2012:707.
6. Collins RD. *Blunting the Double Edge of Corticosteroids: Spartanburg Hospital Bulletin*. March 1975.
7. Collins RD. *What Every Patient Should Know about His Health and His Doctor*. New York: Exposition Press; 1973.
8. Anderson DG, Vaccaro AR. *Decision Making in Spinal Care*. 2nd ed. New York, Stuttgart: Thieme; 2013.

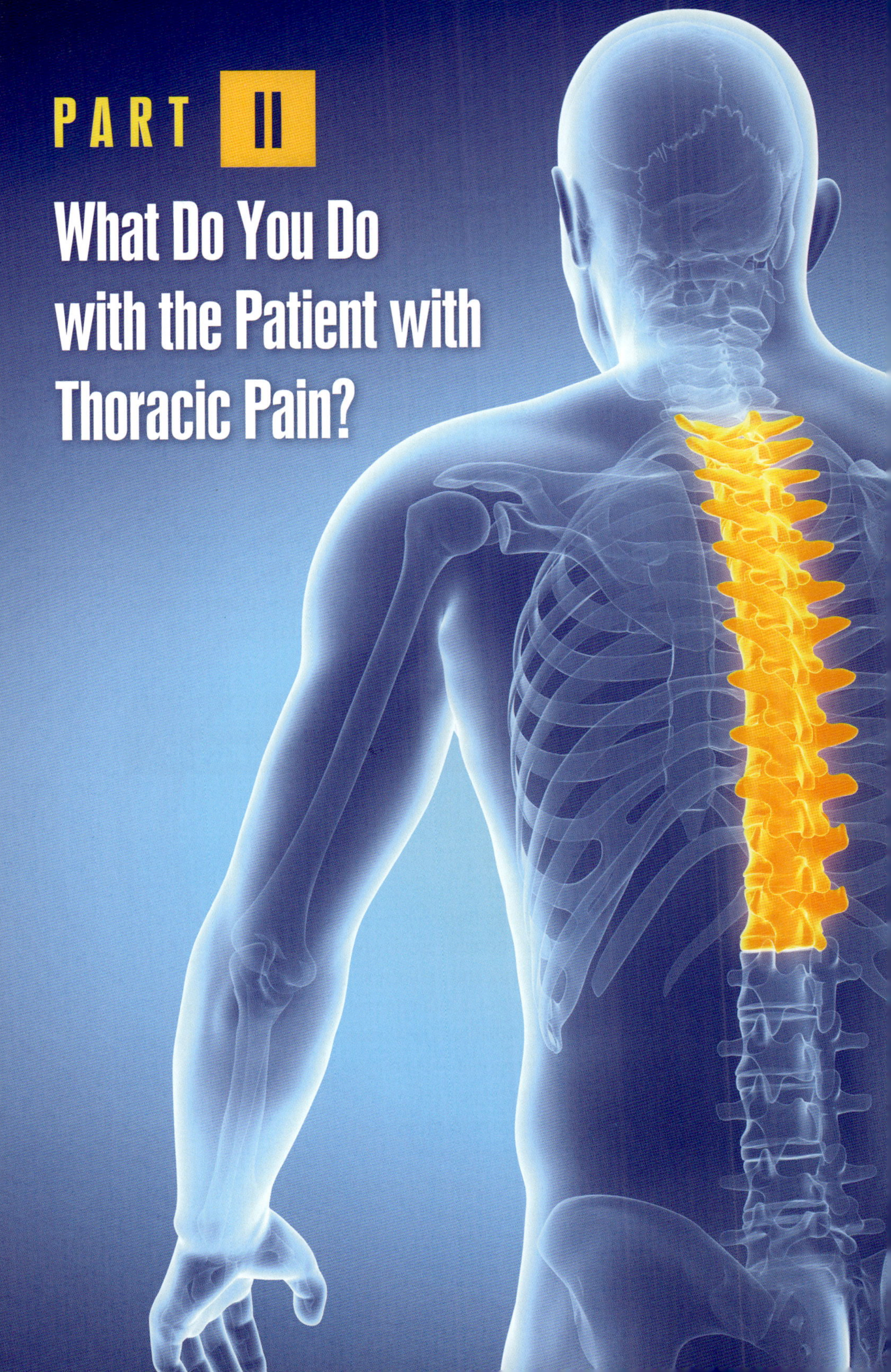
PART II
What Do You Do with the Patient with Thoracic Pain?

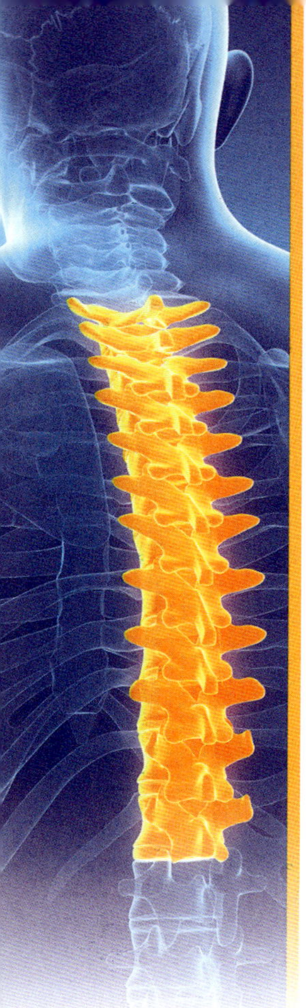

A Taking a History of the Patient with Thoracic Pain

Here again, it is wise to have a list of diagnostic possibilities (Table 2-1 and Figure 2-1) in mind before you begin questioning the patient. We have already explored the use of anatomy in developing such a list, so this time let's use the mnemonic **MINT**, which stands for **M**alformation, **I**nflammation, **N**eoplasm, and **T**rauma.

Malformation would suggest scoliosis. *Inflammation* would suggest an epidural abscess, herpes zoster, pyelonephritis, or pleurisy. *Neoplasm* should suggest primary or metastatic tumors of the spine and lung (mesothelioma, etc.). *Trauma* should suggest fractures, herniated disc (extremely rare), and sprains.

TABLE 2-1

List of the Most Likely Causes of Thoracic Pain

1. Strain, contusions
2. Herpes zoster
3. Scoliosis
4. Fracture
5. Osteoporosis
6. Degenerative spondylosis (osteoarthritis)
7. Primary and metastatic tumor
8. Myocardial infarction or coronary insufficiency
9. Mesothelioma and other pulmonary neoplasms
10. Pneumonia and pleurisy
11. Epidural abscess
12. Rheumatoid spondylosis
13. Pyelonephritis
14. Chronic pancreatitis or pancreatic neoplasm
15. Herniated disc

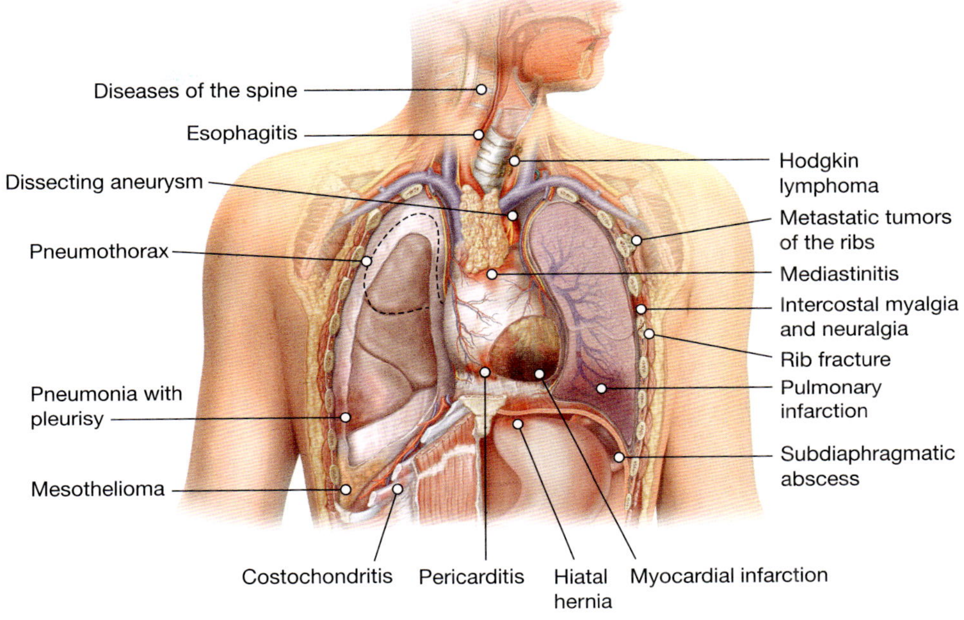

FIGURE 2-1: Illustration of Causes of Thoracic Pain

Onset: Is the thoracic pain *acute*? If so, consider infections (such as epidural abscess, pleurisy, herpes zoster, etc.) and trauma (fracture, sprain, or herniated disc). If the pain followed an injury, you need the details. If it is *chronic*, consider neoplasm (spinal cord tumor, etc.) or congenital and degenerative disorders (scoliosis, osteoporosis, osteoarthritis, etc.).

Back pain may also be referred from acute pancreatitis, cholecystitis, pyelonephritis, myocardial infarction, or dissecting aneurysm.

Associated Symptoms: Fever and chills obviously distinguishes an infectious process while symptoms of weakness, numbness and tingling in the lower extremities, erectile dysfunction, or loss of bladder control would point to a space-occupying lesion of the spinal cord (neoplasm, herniated disc, epidural abscess, etc.). Diaphoresis will point to a myocardial infarction or pulmonary embolism.

Review of Systems: Many of the visceral causes of thoracic pain are illustrated in Figure 2-1.

Hemoptysis suggests a pulmonary embolus or neoplasm while nausea and vomiting prompts consideration of an abdominal condition such as pancreatitis, cholecystitis, or ulcer as well as an inferior wall myocardial infarction. Hematuria frequency or burning on urination would suggest a UTI or renal calculus. We've already discussed the neurologic review of systems under associated symptoms.

Past History: Previous accidents, operations, and hospitalizations should be listed as well as communicable diseases, although tuberculosis of the spinal column is rarely encountered today. If herpes zoster is considered, you will want to ask whether the patient had chickenpox. A history of excessive alcohol consumption may point to pancreatitis, while drug addiction may identify someone feigning illness simply to receive painkillers. To cover all the bases using anatomy as your guide, simply ask the patient if he/she has had heart disease; intestinal disease; kidney disease; skin, joint, or bone disease, etc.

Family History: This may be helpful in cases of scoliosis, or neuromuscular disorders. Once again, the primary objective in the history is to rule out serious conditions that need aggressive action or immediate referral so that you are left with disorders that can be treated conservatively.

B Examination of the Patient with Thoracic Pain

Here again the objective of your examination is to rule out radiculopathy and myelopathy as well as serious conditions such as myocardial infarction, pneumonia with pleurisy, pulmonary embolism, and neoplasms of the lung or pancreas.

Start the examination by observing the patient's gait (Figure 2-2) for spasticity or ataxia that might indicate myelopathy. Perform a Romberg

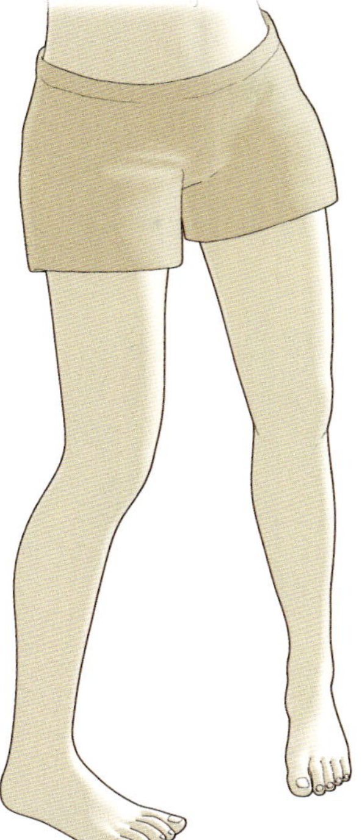

FIGURE 2-2: Gait

test for the same reason (Figure 2-3). Now palpate the paraspinous muscles for muscles spasm or trigger points (Figure 2-4), and while you are at it, look for a rash (herpes zoster). Test range of motion in Lateral Flexion, right and left (Figure 2-5) and Extension and Flexion (Figure 2-6). This will help identify thoracic spondylosis, fractures, and sprains. It may also increase suspicion for less common pathology such as a spinal cord tumor, epidural abscess, or herniated disc. Examine for scoliosis by having the patient bend over and check for protrusions of the scapula on one side or another with the Adams forward bend test (Figure 2-7).[1] Using a pin and cotton applicator or horse hair, examine for dermatomal loss of touch and/or pain that will help identify radiculopathy (Figure 2-8). Check the reflexes (Figure 2-9) and sensation to touch, pain and vibration (Figure 2-10) in the lower extremities. Hyperactive reflexes or diffuse sensory loss would make you suspicious of myelopathy.

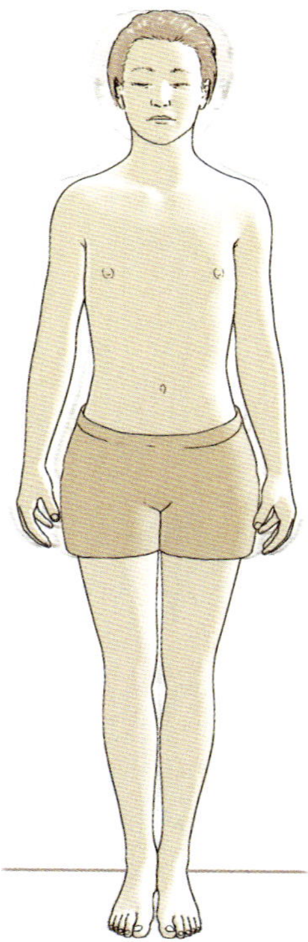

FIGURE 2-3: Romberg

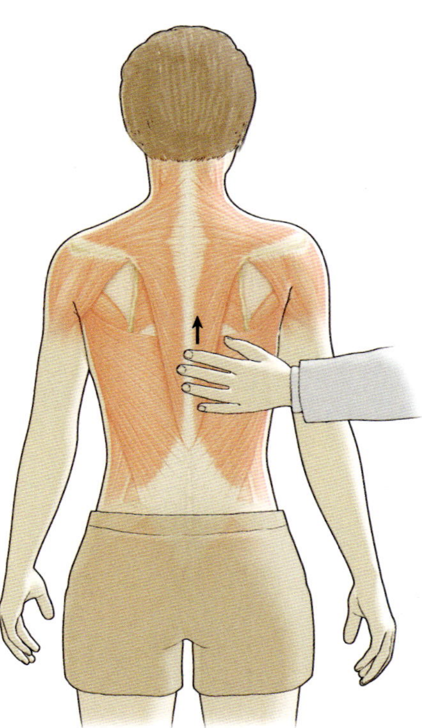

FIGURE 2-4: Palpate for Muscle Spasm and Tenderness

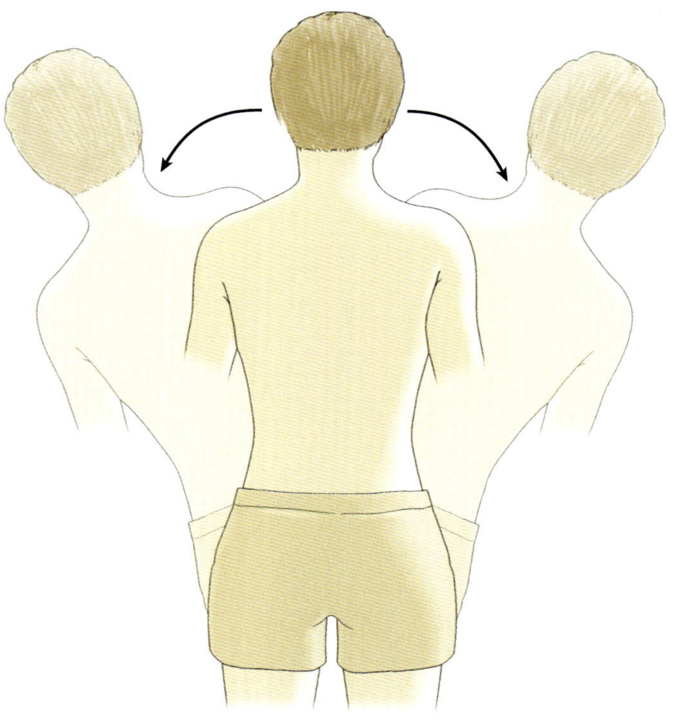

FIGURE 2-5: ROM: Lateral Flexion

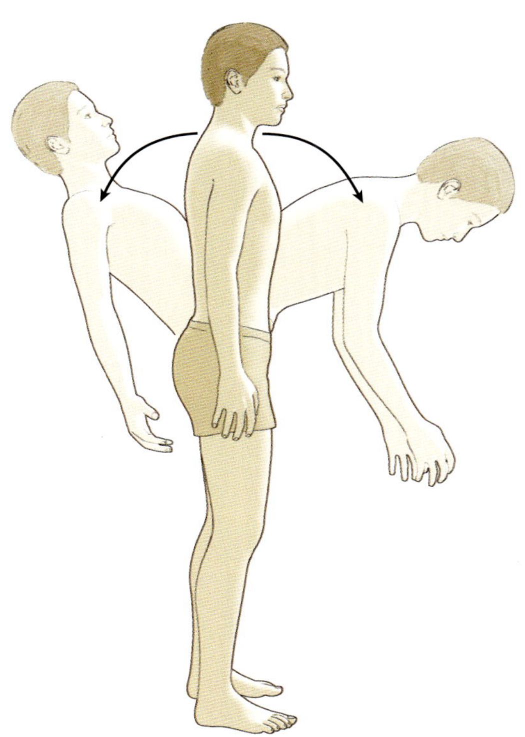

FIGURE 2-6: ROM: Extension and Flexion

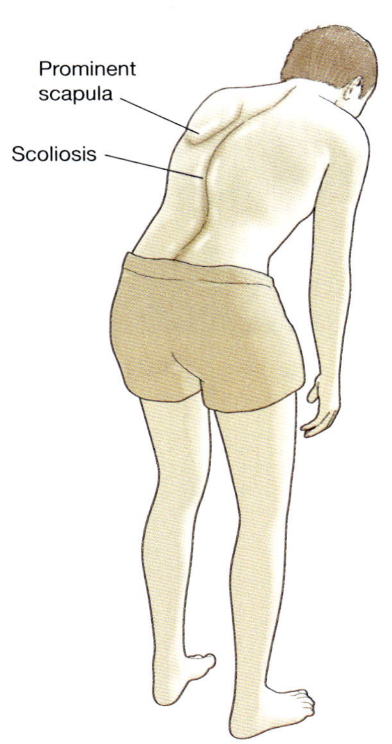

FIGURE 2-7: Examine for Scoliosis

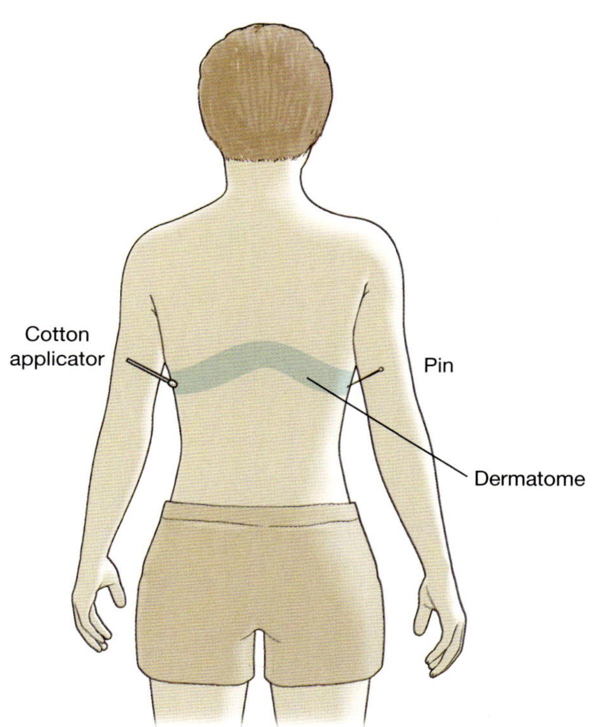

FIGURE 2-8: Test for Dermatomal Sensory Loss

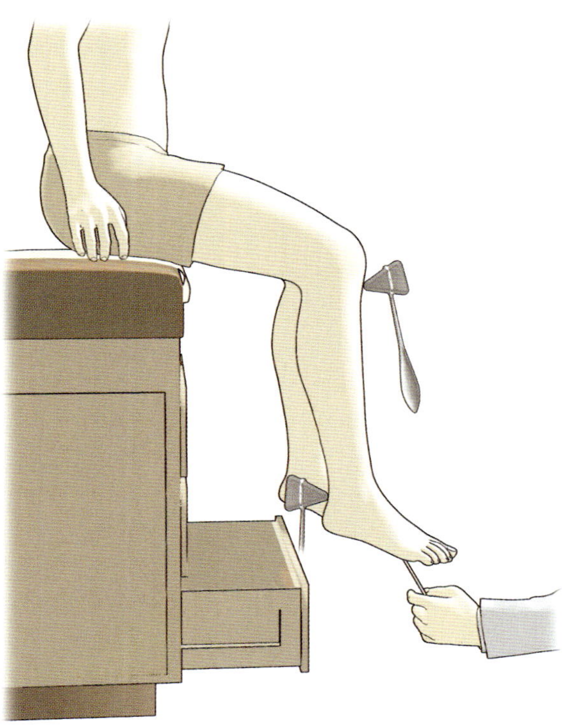

FIGURE 2-9: Reflexes Lower Extremities

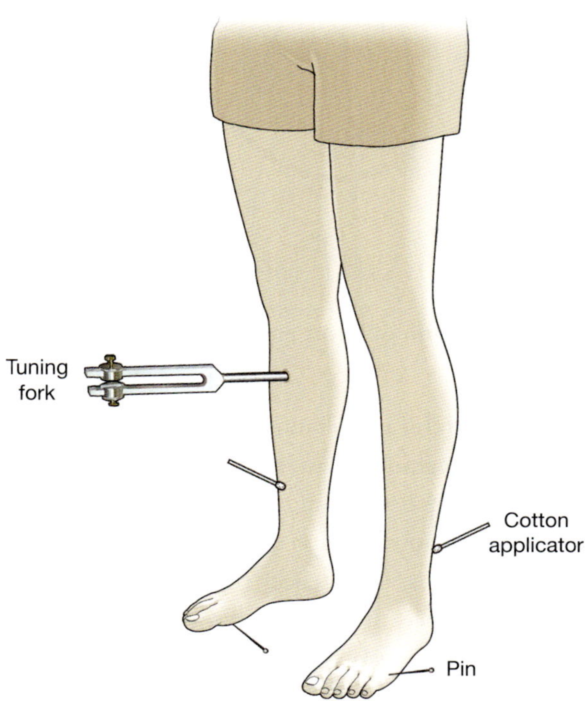

FIGURE 2-10: Sensation in Lower Extremities

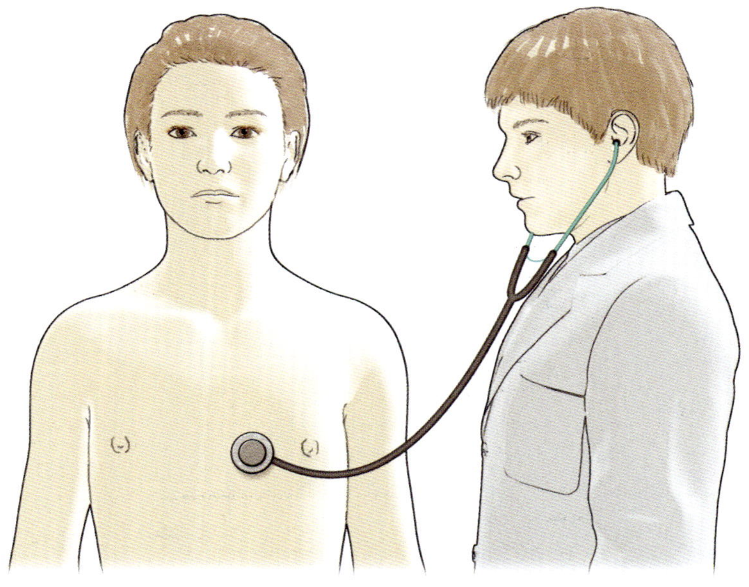

FIGURE 2-11: Auscultation of Heart and Lungs

Finally, perform careful auscultation of the heart and lungs (Figure 2-11) to rule out serious pathology in these organs such as myocardial infarction, pulmonary embolism, and dissecting aneurysm. Of course you should already be suspicious of these disorders based on your history. If a dissecting aneurysm is suspected, check the blood pressure in each upper extremity for a difference. If after the above examination procedures you suspect myelopathy, be sure to do a rectal examination for tone and control.

C Diagnosis of the Patient with Thoracic Pain

When you have finished your history and physical examination, you are presented with four scenarios that will determine your workup and therapeutic options.

1. **Thoracic pain with no radiation, with or without a history of trauma and a normal neurologic and cardiopulmonary exam.** The diagnosis in these cases is most likely a thoracic sprain or spondylosis, but a fracture needs to be ruled out. A CBC, sedimentation rate, chemistry panel, cardiac enzymes, EKG, chest x-ray, and x-ray of the thoracic spine should be ordered before deciding to treat these patients conservatively. If the trauma is severe, perhaps a CT scan is needed to rule out fracture.
2. **Thoracic pain with no history of trauma, no radiation, normal neurologic exam, and abnormalities on the general physical exam.** The diagnosis in these cases includes pulmonary embolism, myocardial infarction, pneumonia, pancreatitis, etc., which may be treated by the primary care provider but often require hospitalization and referral to an appropriate specialist.
3. **Thoracic pain with questionable or mild signs of radiculopathy and no abnormalities on the general physical examination with or without a history of trauma.** Here we must entertain the possibility of a significant compression fracture, herniated disc, epidural abscess, or spinal cord tumor, and the workup includes a CBC, sedimentation rate, chemistry panel, serum protein electrophoresis, chest x-ray, and x-ray of the thoracic spine. If these studies are negative, conservative treatment may be justified, but a neurologic consult may be wise at the onset.
4. **Thoracic pain, with or without a history of trauma with definite signs of radiculopathy and/or myelopathy.** The diagnosis in these cases is usually a compression fracture, herniated disc, epidural abscess, or primary or metastatic neoplasm, and immediate referral to a neurosurgeon is imperative. Ordering special diagnostic procedure such as an MRI or a CT scan may cause an unnecessary delay, and a referral will be made regardless of the outcome. Besides, the specialist is better able to determine what study to order.

D Conservative Management of the Patient with Thoracic Pain

Acute Thoracic Pain: The conservative management of a patient with acute thoracic pain (Table 2-2) begins with nonnarcotic analgesics such as acetaminophen and NSAIDs such as ibuprofen 600 to 800 mg T.I.D. or Naprosyn 250 to 500 mg B.I.D. The NSAIDs should be taken with meals or a large glass of water to avoid an ulcer. Celecoxib and meloxicam have the advantage of being less likely to produce an ulcer or GI bleeding, but unfortunately the television medium has unfairly emphasized that these drugs may cause an MI or a stroke.

TABLE 2-2
Management of Thoracic Pain

Conservative Management

1. Analgesics
2. Nonsteroidal anti-inflammatory drugs
3. Muscle relaxants
4. Corticosteroids
5. Reducing diet
6. Thoracolumbar support
7. Physiotherapy
8. Exercises
9. Trigger point injections
10. Facet injections
11. Antidepressants and anticonvulsants
12. Prayer

Surgical Management

1. Posterolateral transpedicular, transfacet pedicle-sparing costotransversectomy
2. Microendoscopic keyhole diskectomy

Muscle relaxants such as cyclobenzaprine (Flexeril) 10 mg T.I.D. or metaxalone (Skelaxin) 800 mg T.I.D. may be effective, but it is questionable as to whether they are any more useful than a placebo. Adding a short course of corticosteroids such as prednisone 30 mg a day and gradually reducing the dose over a 7- to 10-day period may be helpful, but a course of alternate-day steroids (5 to 20 mg of prednisone) is even more successful in the author's experience.

Narcotics are to be avoided unless they are administered under supervision. If a patient is in such severe pain that continuous narcotics are needed, perhaps the patient should be hospitalized. A thoracolumbar support and a short period of bed rest have also been valuable. If there is point tenderness in the paraspinous muscles, trigger point injections are often effective.

Chronic Thoracic Pain: Initial conservative treatment of chronic thoracic pain is similar to the treatment of acute thoracic pain. However, obese patients need to be put on a reducing diet such as the fruit and vegetable diet already described (Table 1-4). Exercises are also effective. The simplest exercise is to have the patient lie in the recumbent position with arms extended at a 90-degree angle and rotate the arms back and forth while the legs and hips remain stable. Amazing results may be achieved in a few days of doing this exercise 5 to 10 minutes three times a day.

Trigger point and facet injections with or without a corticosteroid are also very effective. There is no need to get the needle into the facet joint. Injection near the joint is just as effective.

Antidepressants such as duloxetine and anticonvulsants such as gabapentin may also be helpful, but if these are contemplated, a referral to a pain management specialist is wise. When pain persists despite conservative therapy, a consult with a neurosurgeon is indicated. Table 2-2 also lists a few of the surgical procedures available. Figure 2-12 depicts an algorithm of the management of the patient with thoracic pain.

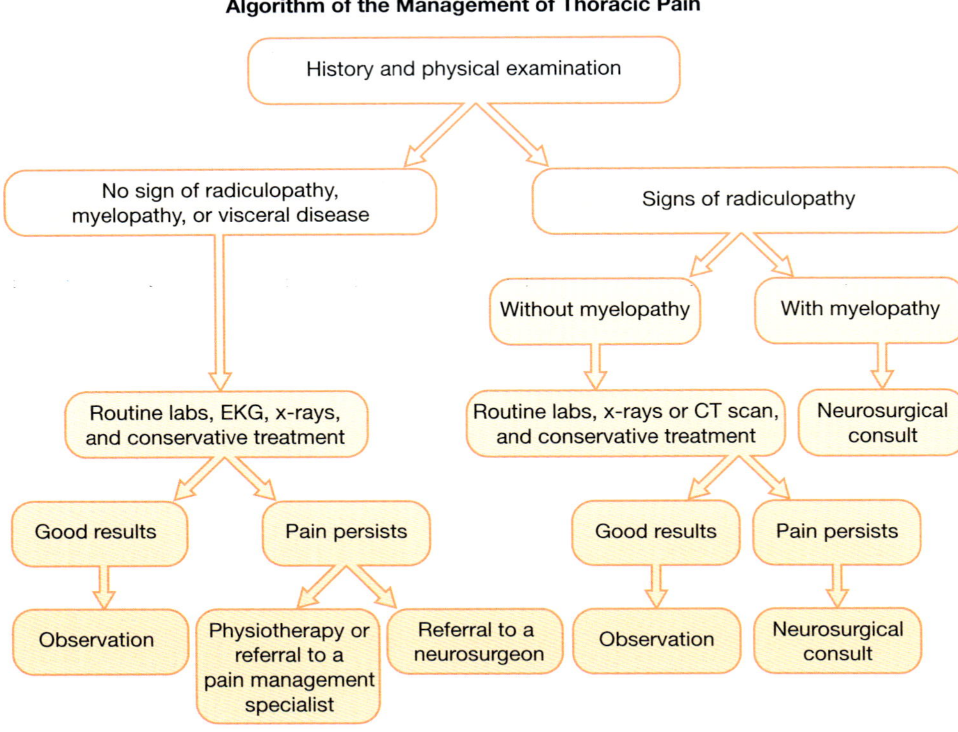

FIGURE 2-12: Management of Thoracic Pain Algorithm

E Illustrated Cases of Thoracic Pain

Normal Anatomy of the Thoracic Spine (Figure 2-13)

Thoracic Sprain (Figure 2-14)

A 29-year-old secretary complained of recurrent pain in her back for several months especially after working at the computer all day. She denied previous injury, and review of systems was unremarkable.

Neurologic examination revealed marked point tenderness at the medial border of the right scapula (point 1) but was otherwise unremarkable. The area was injected with 3 cc of 2% lidocaine, which completely relieved her pain. Subsequent injections with lidocaine and corticosteroids along with exercise and improved posture gave her lasting relief.

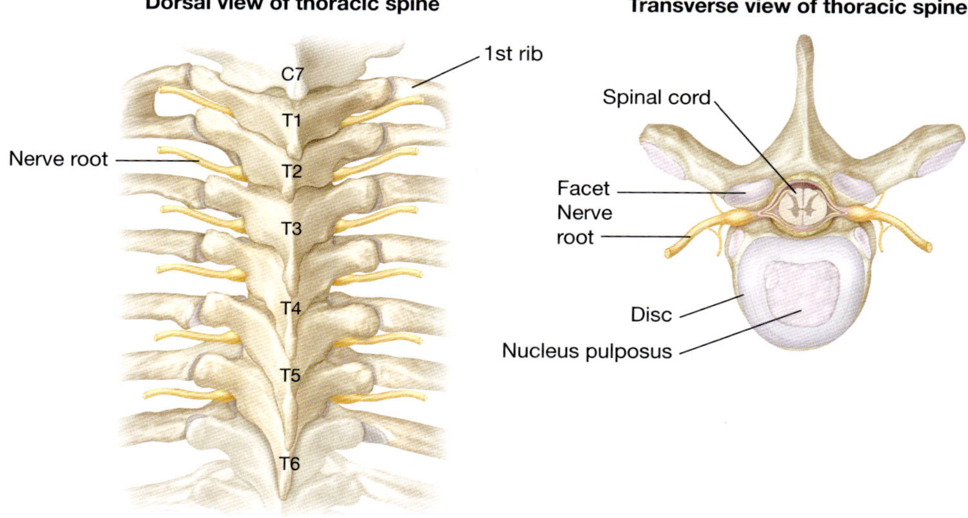

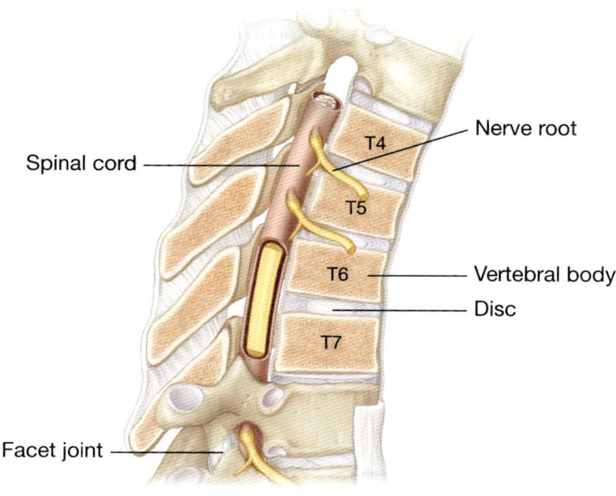

FIGURE 2-13: Normal Anatomy of the Thoracic Spine

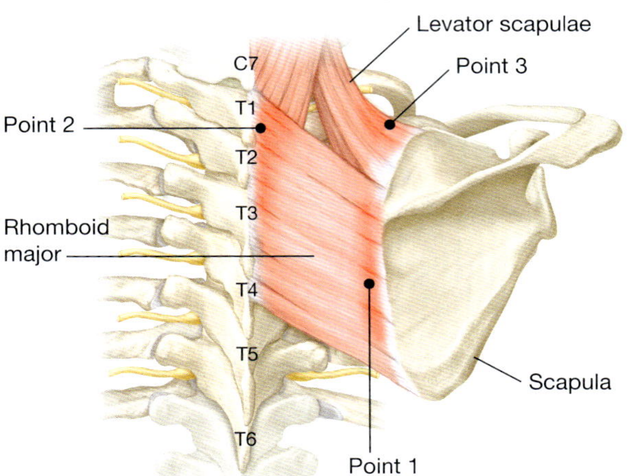

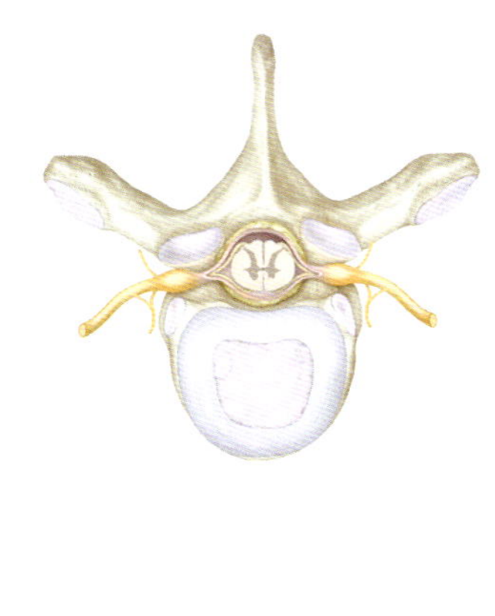

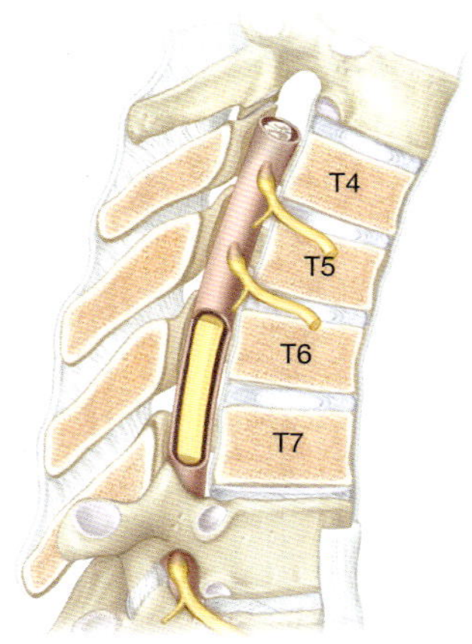

FIGURE 2-14: Thoracic Sprain

Differential Diagnosis

1. Herniated disc
2. Thoracic spondylosis
3. Postherpetic neuralgia
4. Spinal cord tumor
5. Scoliosis
6. Compression fracture
7. Cervical sprain

Discussion: The author has found that many cases of chronic upper back pain respond to trigger point injections especially in young people. Two other areas that almost uniformly respond are in the subtrapezius area at T1 (Point 2) and the insertion of the levator scapular muscle (Point 3).

Herpes Zoster (Figure 2-15)

A 72-year-old white male complained of severe constant scapular pain radiating to his axilla and right side of his chest. He denied shortness of breath or diaphoresis. Past history revealed he had chickenpox as a child.

Neurologic examination was unremarkable except for a vesicular rash in the distribution of his right 5th thoracic nerve. Laboratory and x-ray examinations were unremarkable.

Differential Diagnosis

1. Pulmonary embolism
2. Coronary insufficiency
3. Pneumothorax
4. Epidemic myalgia
5. Thoracic spondylosis
6. Herniated thoracic disc
7. Compression fracture

Treatment with valacyclovir, 1,000 mg T.I.D. and analgesics was successful.

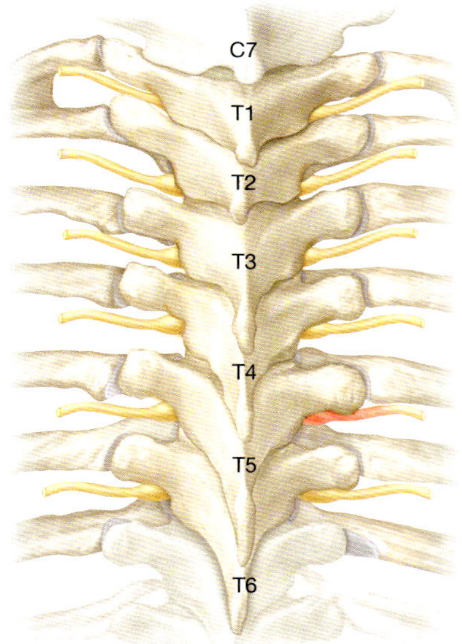

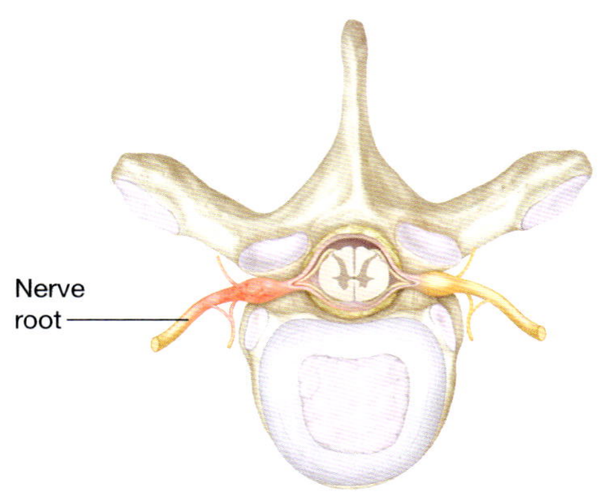

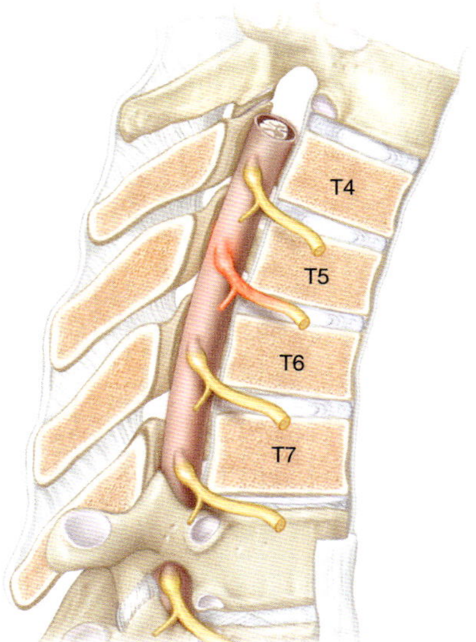

FIGURE 2-15: Herpes Zoster

Discussion: The vesicular rash makes this diagnosis simple, but often it is not present especially at the initial visit. Serious conditions such as myocardial or pulmonary infarction must always be ruled out. Zoster vaccine (Zostavax) should be given to all patients over 50 years of age.

Herniated Thoracic Disc (Figure 2-16)

A 20-year-old black male college football player presented to the ER with severe constant upper back and right chest pain that began after being tackled during a game. The pain was increased by coughing and extension and lateral flexion of his spine. Review of systems revealed no SOB or other respiratory or cardiac symptoms.

Past History was unremarkable.

Neurologic examination revealed loss of sensation in his right T5 dermatome, but power and sensation were intact on all four extremities and deep tendon reflexes were symmetrical. There were no pathologic reflexes.

An MRI of the thoracic spine revealed a lateral disc herniation at T5-T6 compressing the T6 nerve root.

Conservative Treatment with NSAID's and physical therapy alleviated most of his pain, but he was restricted from playing football for the rest of the season.

Differential Diagnosis

1. Thoracic sprain
2. Compression fracture
3. Pneumothorax
4. Herpes zoster

Discussion: A large number of these cases present with symptoms and signs of myelopathy, so a consult with a neurologist or neurosurgeon is wise. It is also important to do a thorough medical workup to rule out cardiac or pulmonary pathology especially in patients who present with no significant history of trauma.

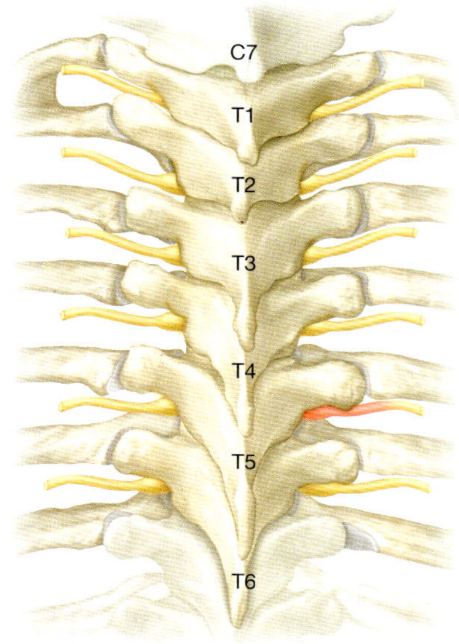

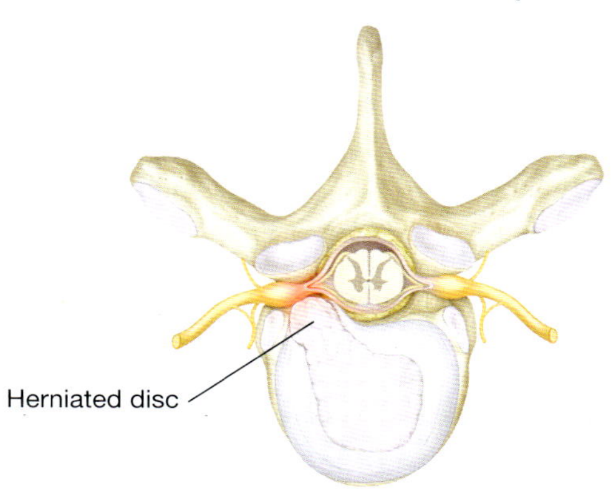

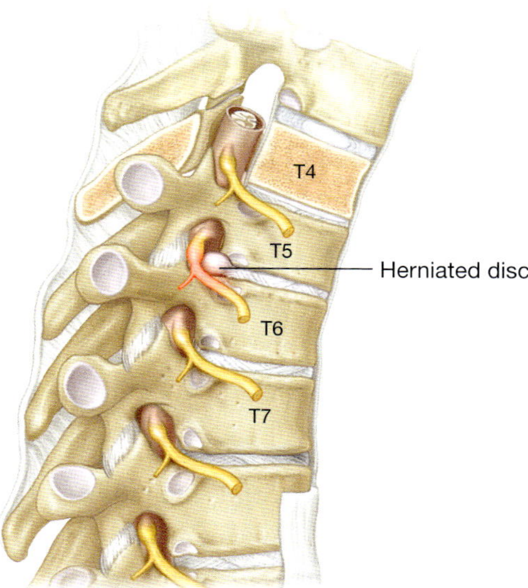

FIGURE 2-16: Herniated Thoracic Disc

Neoplasm of the Thoracic Spine (Figure 2-17)

A 64-year-old white female had been treated for anemia by her local physician for several years. Six months prior to admission she developed mild girdle-like pain in her upper back radiating to her breasts bilaterally. Three months prior to admission, she developed weakness and numbness and tingling in her legs. By the time she was admitted to the neurosurgical service, she was in a wheel chair and had occasional urinary and fecal incontinence.

Neurologic examination revealed hyperactive reflexes, loss of vibratory and position sense in her lower extremities, and a sensory level at T5 bilaterally. There were bilateral Babinski signs.

Laboratory examination showed a normochromic, normocytic anemia and elevated gamma globulin on serum protein electrophoresis, and her urine was positive for Bence Jones protein.

x-Ray of the thoracic spine revealed osteolytic punched-out lesions and diffuse osteopenia. MRI demonstrated a prominent mass at T5 that on surgery proved to be a plasmacytoma.

Differential Diagnosis

1. Other primary and metastatic tumors
2. Epidural abscess
3. Compression fracture
4. Herniated disc
5. Multiple sclerosis
6. Pernicious anemia
7. Anterior spinal artery occlusion

Comment: The gradual onset of symptoms is typical of spinal cord tumors, most of which occur in the thoracic area. Any patient with gradual onset of weakness in the lower extremities needs to have a serum protein electrophoresis included in the workup.

Dorsal view of thoracic spine

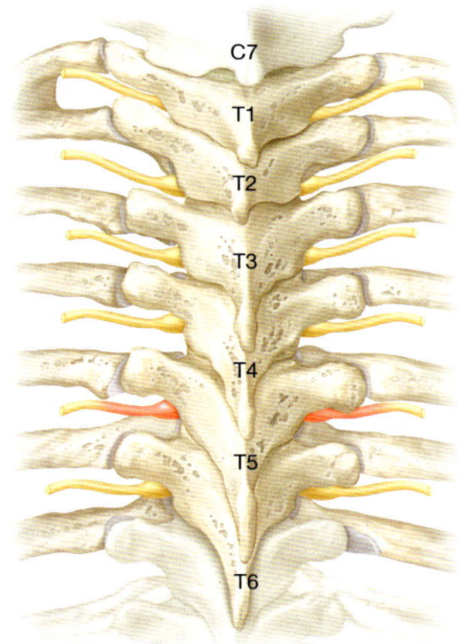

Transverse view of thoracic spine

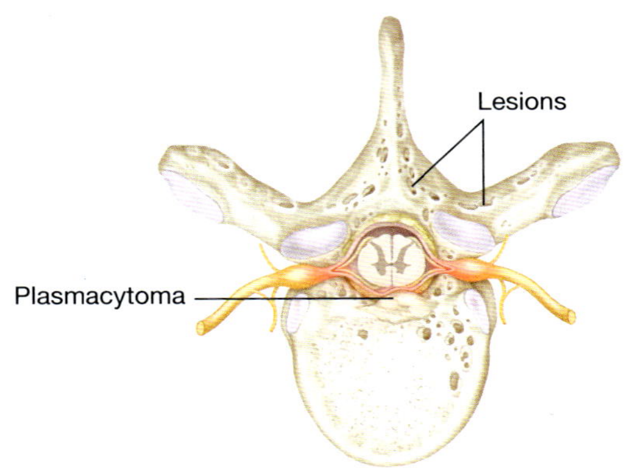

Sagittal view of thoracic spine

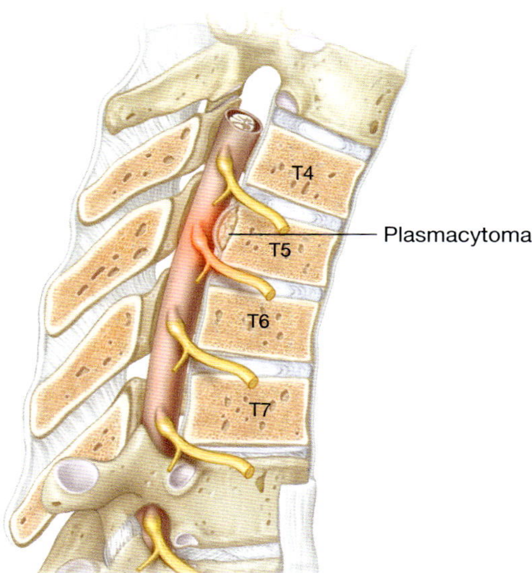

FIGURE 2-17: Neoplasm of the Thoracic Spine

Osteoporosis with Compression Fracture of the Thoracic Spine (Figure 2-18)

A 67-year-old Hispanic female presented to the outpatient clinic with acute upper back pain that developed after lifting furniture. The pain was increased by coughing and sneezing. Past history was unremarkable except that she had been on a reducing diet the past 6 months and lost 60 lbs.

General Physical Examination revealed marked tenderness and paraspinous muscles spasm in the mid thoracic region and thoracic kyphosis, but neurologic examination was unremarkable.

Plain Films of the thoracic spine showed a wedge fracture at T6 and mild osteoporosis. A DXA scan (dual-energy x-ray absorptiometry) was below 2.5 standard deviations of young adult peak mean value. Routine laboratory tests were unremarkable.

Treatment: The patient was started on calcium and vitamin D_3 supplements, and alendronate 10 mg daily.

Differential Diagnosis

1. Menopause
2. Multiple myeloma
3. Hyperthyroidism
4. Malabsorption syndrome
5. Metastatic neoplasm
6. Thoracic spondylosis
7. Prolonged corticosteroid use
8. Hyperparathyroidism

Discussion: Spontaneous fractures of the thoracic spine are almost always related to osteoporosis, but metastatic carcinoma and multiple myelomas should always be considered. Newer therapy with the bisphosphonates has become the mainstay of prevention and treatment,

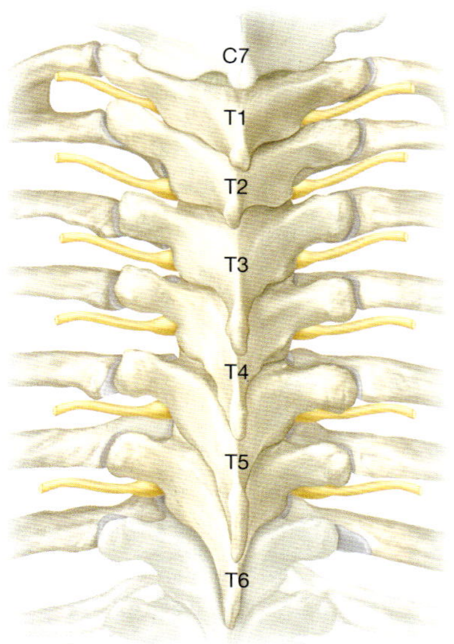

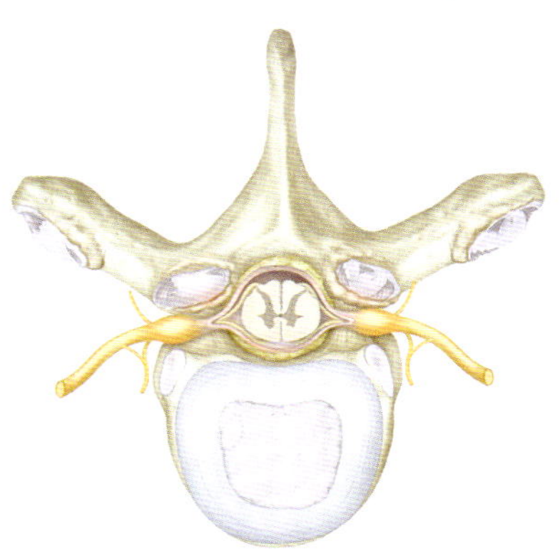

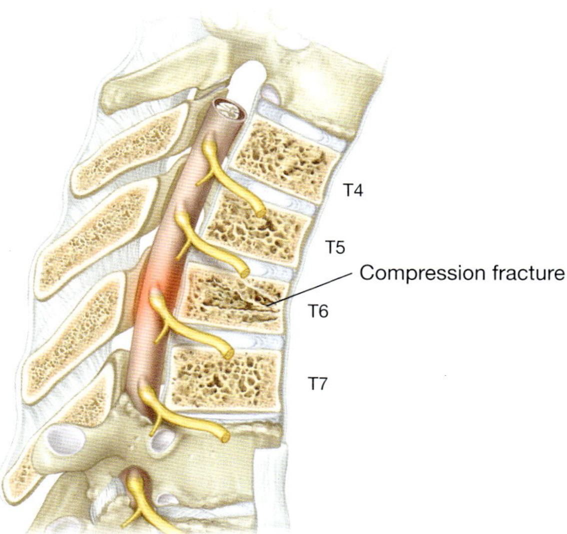

FIGURE 2-18: Osteoporosis with Compression Fracture of the Thoracic Spine

but hormone replacement therapy is still recommended if there are menopausal symptoms and no history of breast cancer in the patient or her family. All patients should receive a vitamin D_3 supplement of 2,000 units a day.

Epidural Abscess (Figure 2-19)

A 58-year-old diabetic female developed fever, severe thoracic and girdle-like pain around her chest on her way to work. By the time she arrived at the emergency room, she had weakness in both legs and incontinence.

Neurologic examination revealed weakness, diminished vibratory and position sense, and positive Babinski signs in both lower extremities. Deep tendon reflexes were symmetrically depressed. There was loss of pain and touch to the level of T6 bilaterally.

Routine laboratory examination showed a white count of 23,000 and increased WBCs and bacteria in her urine. An MRI with gadolinium enhancement demonstrated an abscess at T6.

Treatment with surgical decompression and systemic antibiotics was successful, but it took several months before substantial neurologic recovery was achieved.

Differential Diagnosis

1. Compression fracture
2. Osteomyelitis
3. Spinal cord tumor
4. Multiple sclerosis
5. Pneumonia with pleurisy
6. Tuberculosis
7. Dissecting aneurysm

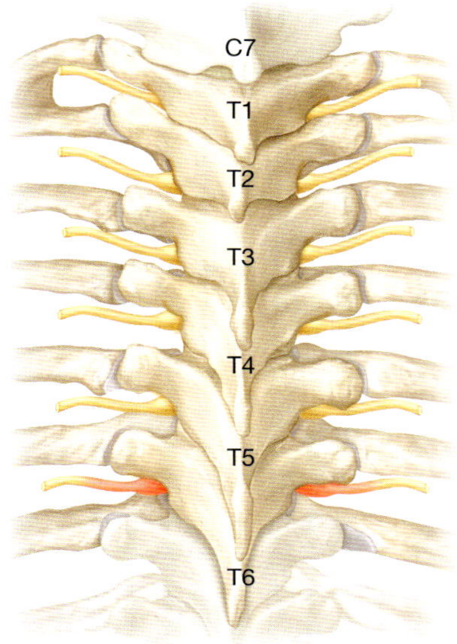

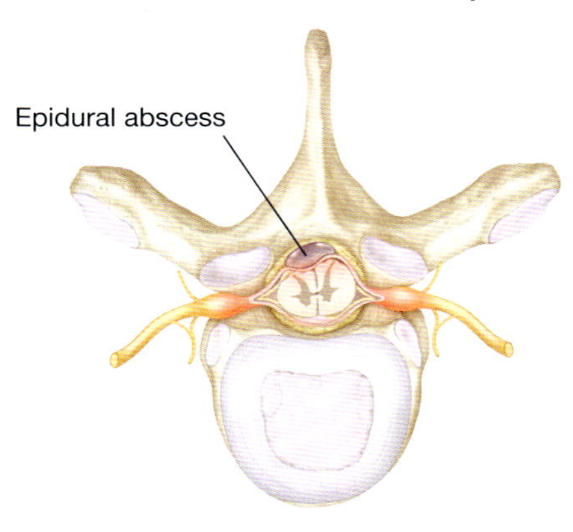

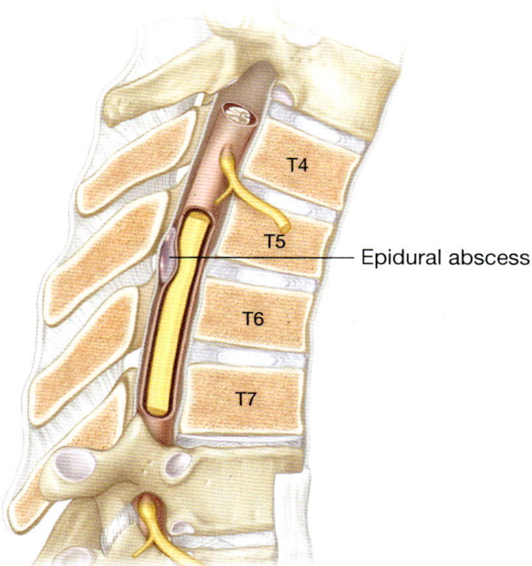

FIGURE 2-19: Epidural Abscess

Discussion: This condition must be considered in anyone with acute thoracic pain, fever, and chills, especially a diabetic. It is a medical emergency.

REFERENCE

1. Anderson DG, Vaccaro AR. *Decision Making in Spinal Care*. 2nd ed. New York, NY: Thieme; 2013.

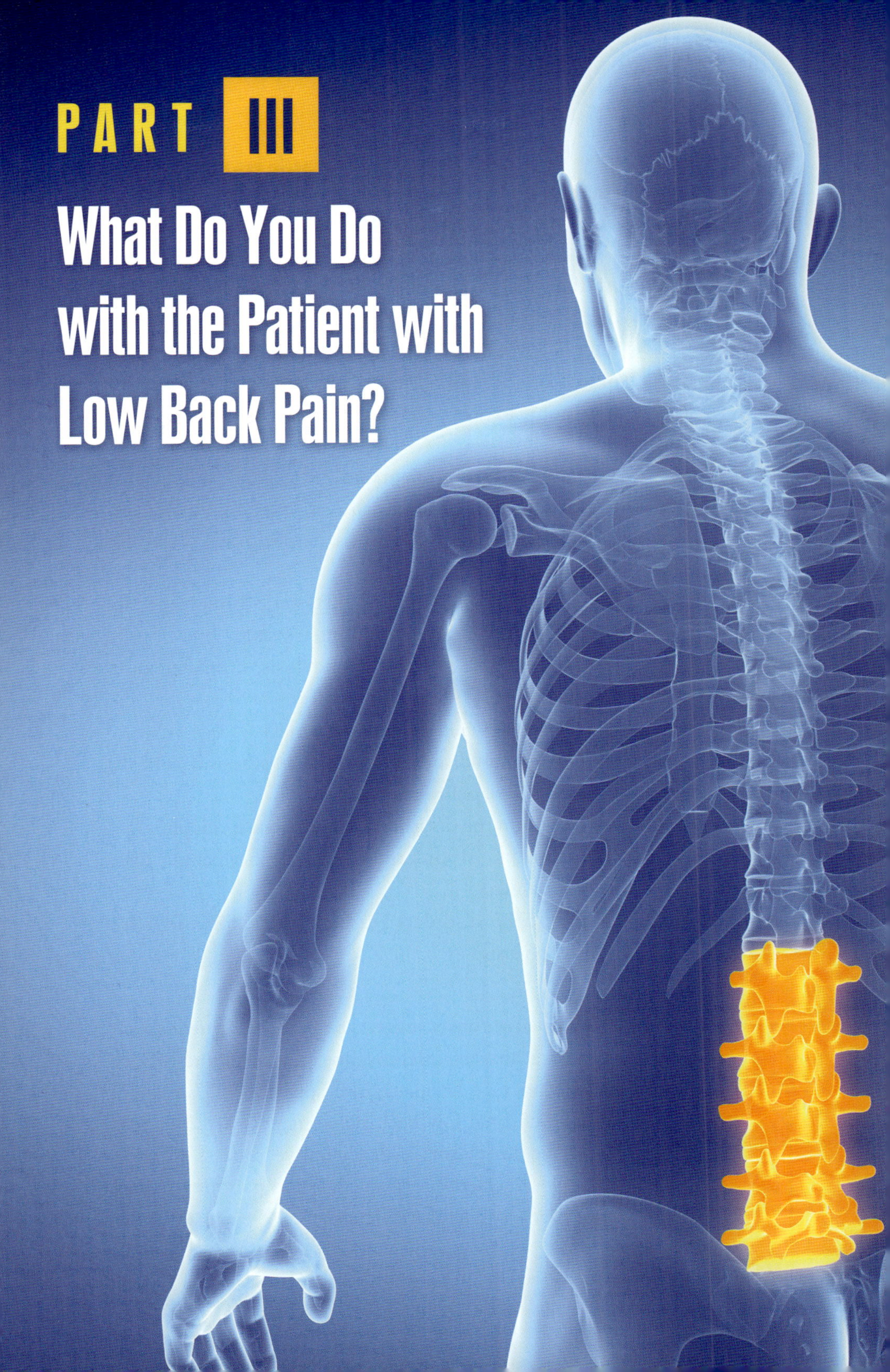
PART III
What Do You Do
with the Patient with
Low Back Pain?

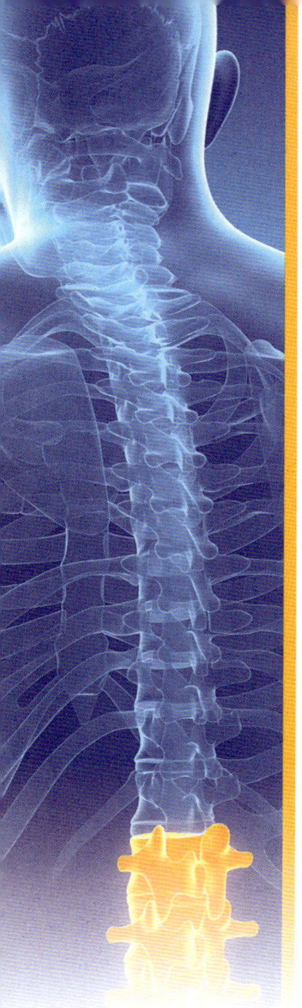

A Taking a History of the Patient with Low Back Pain

At the risk of repetition of the points made in the discussion of neck and thoracic pain, don't start your interview until you have a list of diagnostic possibilities in mind (Table 3-1 and Figures 3-1 and 3-2). Another excellent mnemonic to help you with this is VINDICATE:

V—Vascular (aortic aneurysm)
I—Inflammation (epidural abscess, osteomyelitis, sacroiliitis, rheumatoid spondylosis, herpes zoster, prostatitis, PID, etc.)
N—Neoplasm (primary or metastatic tumors of the spine, ovarian tumors, endometriosis)
D—Degenerative (lumbar spondylosis, herniated disc, osteoporosis)
I—Intoxication (radiculoneuropathies)
C—Congenital disorders (spondylolisthesis, scoliosis, spina bifida, ochronosis, etc.)
A—Autoimmune disorders (rheumatoid spondylitis)
T—Traumatic disorders (fracture, herniated disc, sprains, etc.)
E—Endocrine disorders (diabetic radiculoneuropathy, osteoporosis)

Onset: An acute onset suggests an infectious process such as epidural abscess, osteomyelitis, prostatitis and PID, or trauma (fracture, herniated disc, sprain), while a gradual onset of chronic low back pain suggests a primary or metastatic neoplasm or degenerative process (lumbar spondylosis, osteoporosis, etc.). If the pain began after an accident, you need the details.

TABLE 3-1

List of most Likely Causes of Low Back Pain

1. Sprain, contusion
2. Herniated disc
3. Facet syndrome
4. Degenerative spondylosis (osteoarthritis)
5. Spinal stenosis
6. Fractures
7. Osteoporosis with compression fracture
8. Rheumatoid spondylitis
9. Idiopathic sacroiliitis
10. Osteomyelitis
11. Epidural abscess
12. Primary and metastatic tumors
13. Scoliosis
14. Spondylolisthesis
15. Abdominal aortic aneurysm
16. Prostatitis
17. Pelvic inflammatory disease
18. Endometriosis
19. Pelvic tumors (ovarian cysts, etc.)
20. Litigation
21. Conversion or somatization reaction
22. Fibromyositis

Radiation of the Pain: Radiation of the pain to the buttocks or extremities would suggest a space-occupying lesion such as herniated disc, epidural abscess, or neoplasm.

Aggravation Relief or Precipitation of the Pain: Aggravation of the pain on flexion might suggest a herniated disc, while aggravation on extension would suggest a facet syndrome from spondylosis (osteoarthritis). If the pain persists while lying down, you must consider a neoplasm. Precipitation of the pain in the hips or extremities on walking a certain

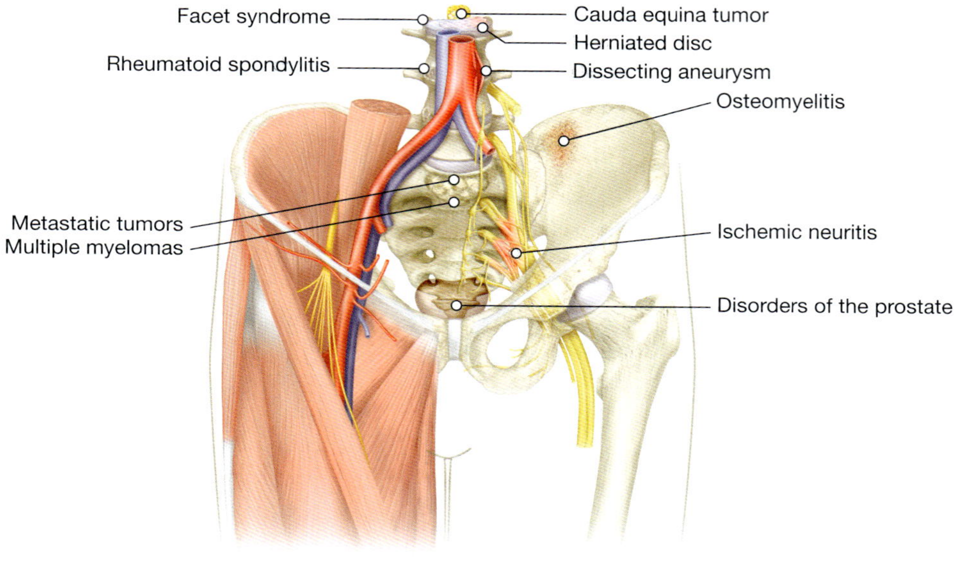

FIGURE 3-1: Illustration of Causes of Low Back Pain

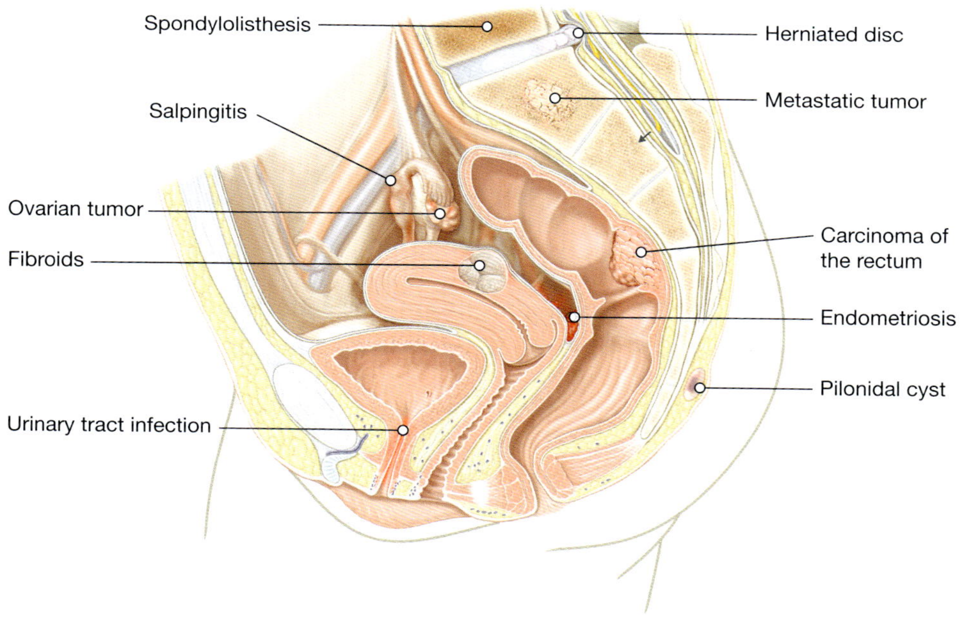

FIGURE 3-2: Illustration of Causes of Low Back Pain

distance suggests neurogenic or vascular claudication. Aggravation of the pain on coughing, sneezing, or straining during a bowel movement would suggest a herniated disc or other space-occupying lesion.

Associated Symptoms: Fever or chills suggest an infectious process such as an epidural abscess, osteomyelitis, prostatitis, or PID. Painful intercourse or irregular menses suggests PID or endometriosis as well as other pelvic pathology. Weakness, paresthesias of the extremities, or gait disturbances point to a radiculopathy. When these symptoms are combined with difficulty voiding or loss of bladder control, one must consider a cauda equina syndrome.

Review of Systems: A careful review of systems is helpful but can be simplified by asking the following questions:

1. Is there pain anywhere else?
2. Is there bleeding from any body orifice?
3. Is there a discharge from any body orifice?
4. Is there a lump or bump anywhere?
5. Is there dysfunction of any organ system? (Difficulty swallowing, breathing, having an erection, indigestion, hearing, seeing, moving your bowels, voiding, walking, etc.).

Past History: Ask about recent or past injuries or accidents, surgeries or hospitalizations. Is there a history of heart disease, lung disease, liver disease, kidney disease, intestinal disease, neurologic disease, or skin, bone, or joint disease? Don't forget psychiatric disease, drug or alcohol addiction, and pending litigation.

Family History: A family history of diabetes, scoliosis, or neuromuscular disorder is important.

Summary: Again it is important to emphasize that just like with neck and thoracic pain the object of the history is to determine if you, the primary care provider, can treat the patient with low back pain conservatively or need to make a referral for more aggressive action.

B Examination of the Patient with Low Back Pain

The examination of the patient with back pain need not take a lot of time. With a little practice, it can be accomplished in 10 to 15 minutes.

Begin the exam by having the patient walk normally back and forth in the exam room. Look for a steppage gait or footdrop or a limp. Have the patient walk on his/her heels (Figure 3-3), which may demonstrate weakness of dorsiflexion of the foot and toes indicating an L5 radiculopathy or peroneal neuropathy. Next, have the patient walk on his/her toes (Figure 3-4). This may indicate an S1 radiculopathy. Then have the patient

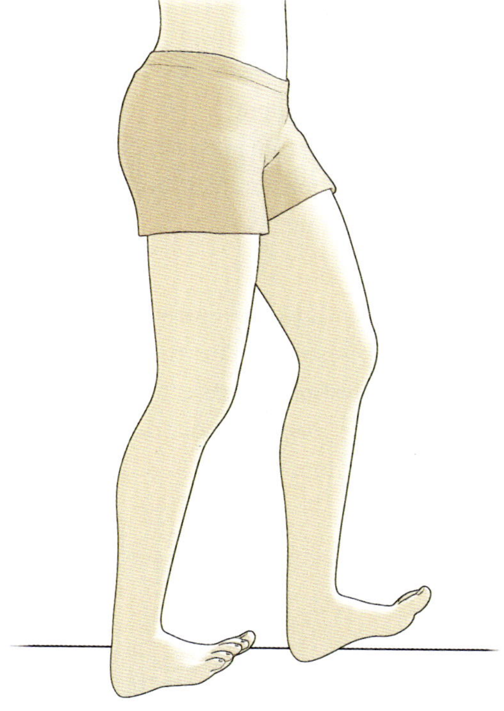

FIGURE 3-3: "Walk On Your Heels"

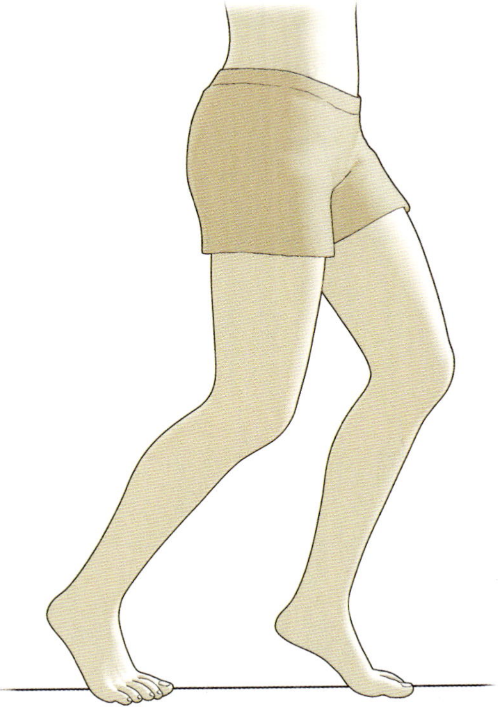

FIGURE 3-4: "Walk On Your Toes"

stand at ease with the legs 12 inches apart and palpate the erector spinae muscles for muscle spasm (Figure 3-5). Normally the muscles will be soft and doughty, but in lumbosacral spine pathology, they can be mildly tight or stiff as a board unilaterally or bilaterally.

Test the range of motion of the lumbar spine by having the patient bend over as far as he or she can before experiencing pain (Figure 3-6) and then extending to the point of pain (Figure 3-7). Normally, patients can extend 25 degrees and bend 75 to 90 degrees. Lateral bending should also be tested (Figure 3-8). This is normally 25 to 30 degrees.

Now, have the patient sit on the end of the exam table and perform straight leg raising (Figure 3-9). Normally there should be no leg pain or restriction to 80 to 90 degrees unless there are short hamstrings. If the patient experiences only an increase in low back pain, the test is negative. Next, have the patient lie down and perform the same maneuver (Figure 3-10).

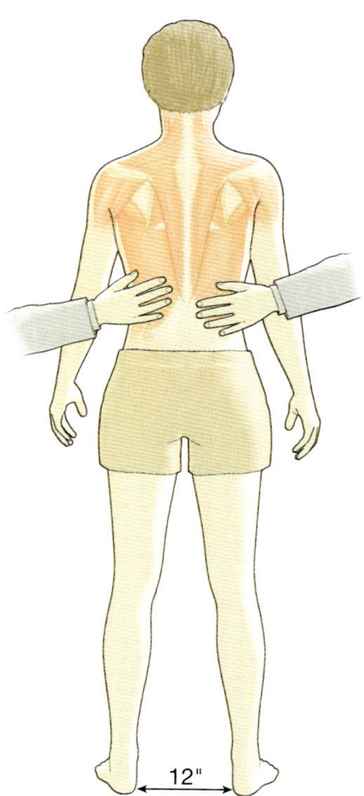

FIGURE 3-5: Palpate for Muscle Spasm

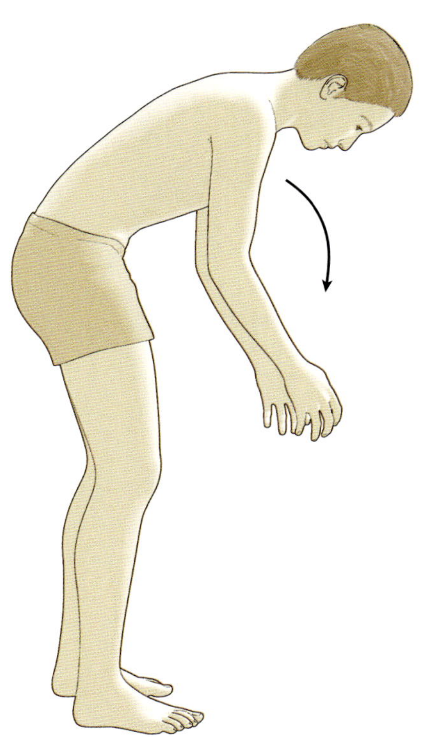

FIGURE 3-6: ROM Flexion

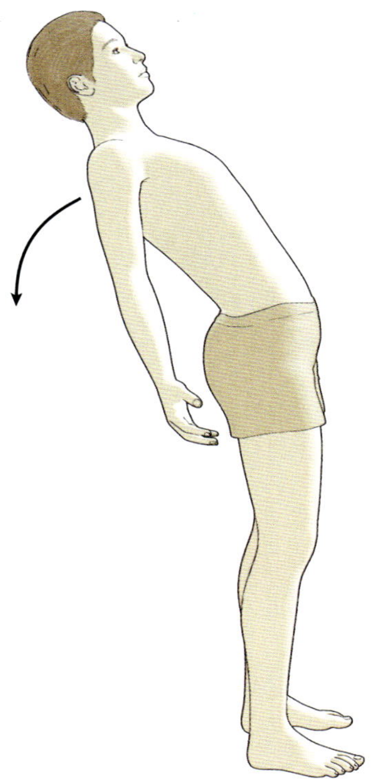

FIGURE 3-7: ROM Extension

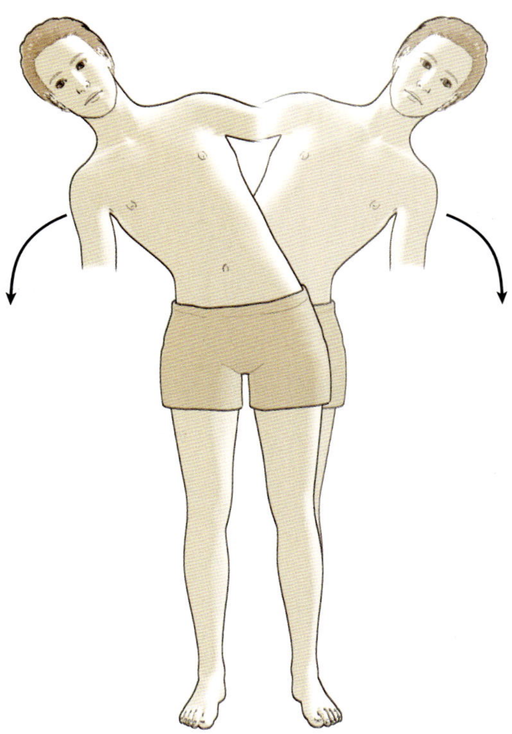

FIGURE 3-8: ROM Lateral Bending

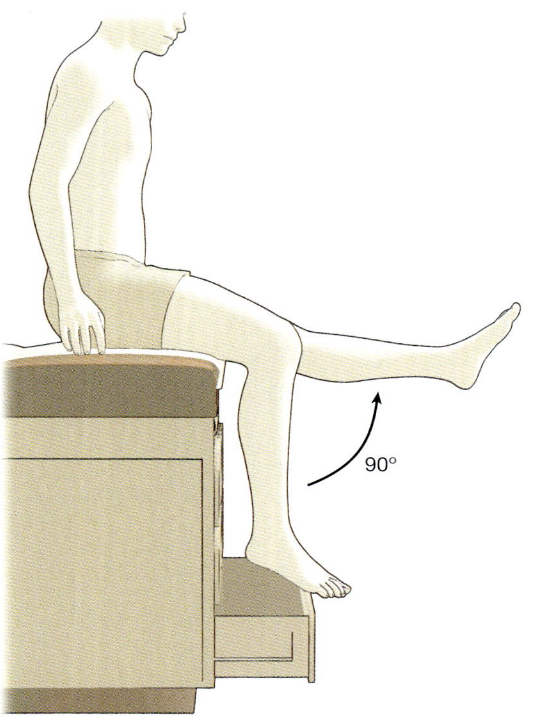

FIGURE 3-9: SLR Sitting

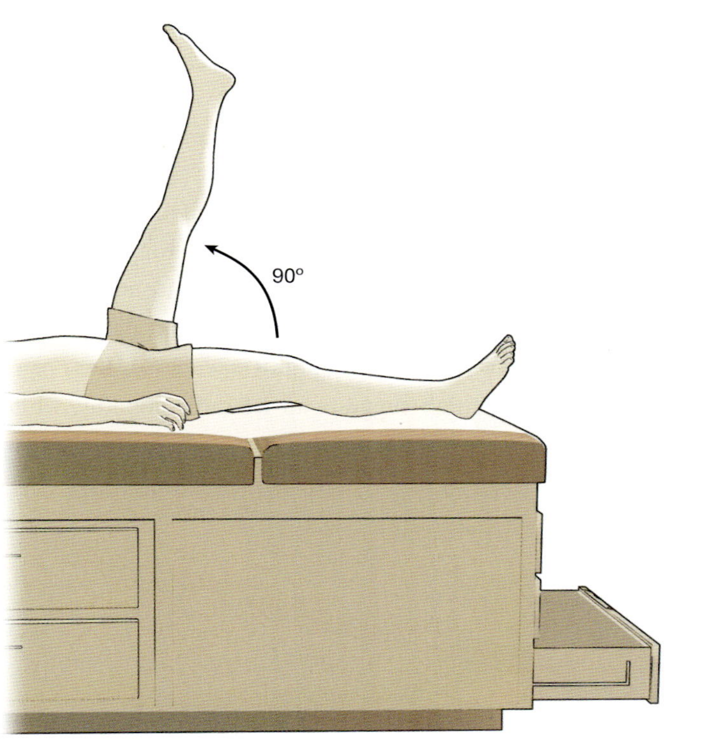

FIGURE 3-10: SLR Lying Down

If he/she is malingering, leg pain may only be experienced in the recumbent position. This is a good place to check for a short leg by simply having the patient stretch the legs out together and observing whether the heels appear at equal length or medial malleoli touch. If there is any doubt, measure the distance between the anterior superior iliac spine and the medial malleolus on each leg (Figure 3-11).

Confirm your findings on the SLR by performing a Lasègue sign (Figure 3-12). Next, perform the femoral stretch on each leg (Figure 3-13) Anterior-thigh pain or resistance anywhere before 80 to 90 degrees may indicate an L3 or L4 radiculopathy.

Test sensation to touch and pain on the big and little toes on each foot and compare the results by testing back and forth (Figure 3-14). The lateral and medial surfaces of the feet may be substituted if there are calluses. Loss of sensation to touch and or pain on the big toe may indicate an L5 radiculopathy, while loss on the little toe may indicate an S1 radiculopathy.

In like manner, test the sensation to touch and pain on the medial and lateral surfaces of the anterior thigh (Figure 3-15). Loss of sensation over the anterolateral thigh suggests an L4 radiculopathy, while loss of

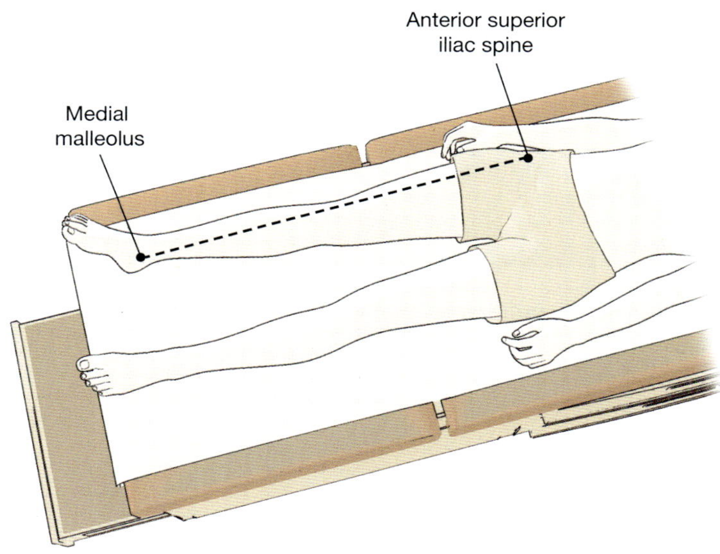

FIGURE 3-11: Measure Leg Length

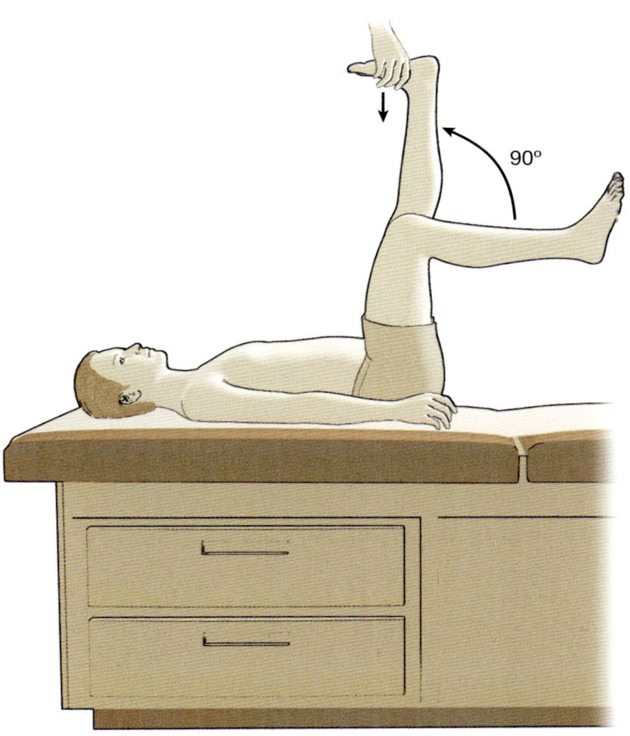

FIGURE 3-12: Lasègue Sign

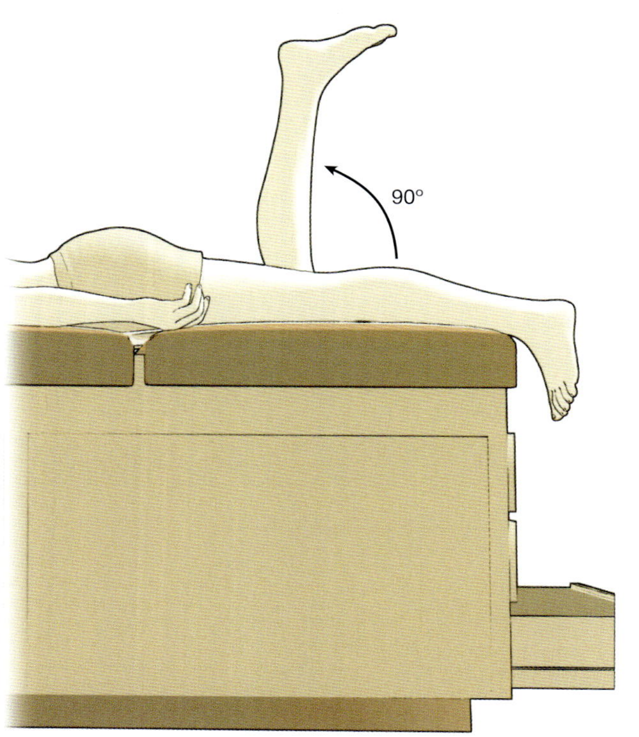

FIGURE 3-13: Femoral Stretch Test

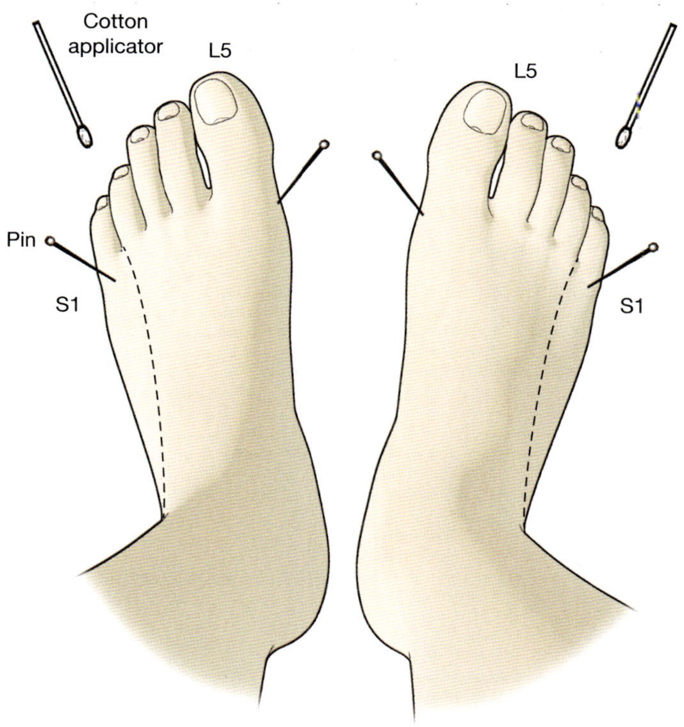

FIGURE 3-14: Test Sensation L5-S1 Dermatome

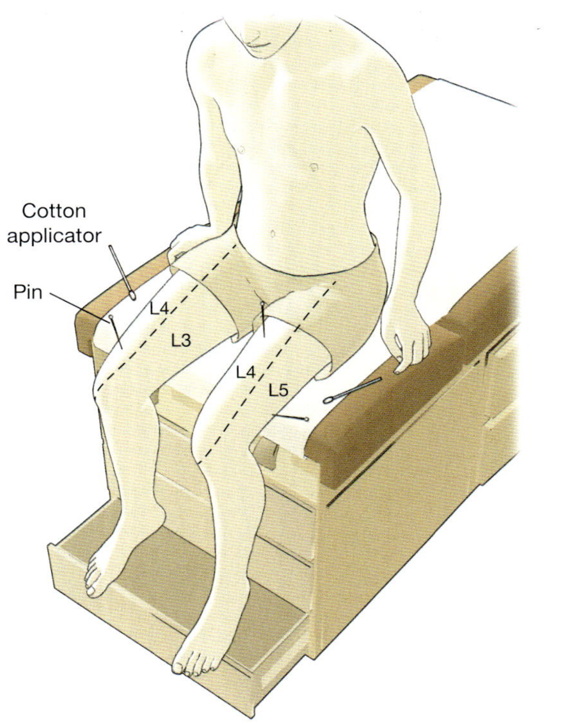

FIGURE 3-15: Test Sensation L3-L4 Dermatome

sensation over the anteromedial surface may indicate an L3 radiculopathy. If a cauda equina lesion is suspected, test the sensation over the sacrum (Figure 3-16).

Next, we need to assess muscle power. Check the power of dorsiflexion of the toes and feet (Figure 3-17) on each extremity and note any difference. Weakness of dorsiflexion of the big toe is almost always due to an L5 radiculopathy or peroneal neuropathy. In like manner, check the power of extension (or plantar flexion) of the foot and toes (Figure 3-18).

Move on to testing the power of knee flexion (Figure 3-19) and extension (Figure 3-20). Note any difference. Weakness on extension is often an indication of L4 radiculopathy.

The deep tendon reflexes are next tested at the knee and ankle and checked for comparison (Figure 3-21). An absent ankle jerk on one extremity is strong evidence of an S1 radiculopathy, while a diminished ankle jerk may indicate an L5 or S1 radiculopathy. A diminished knee jerk on one lower extremity suggests an L4 radiculopathy.

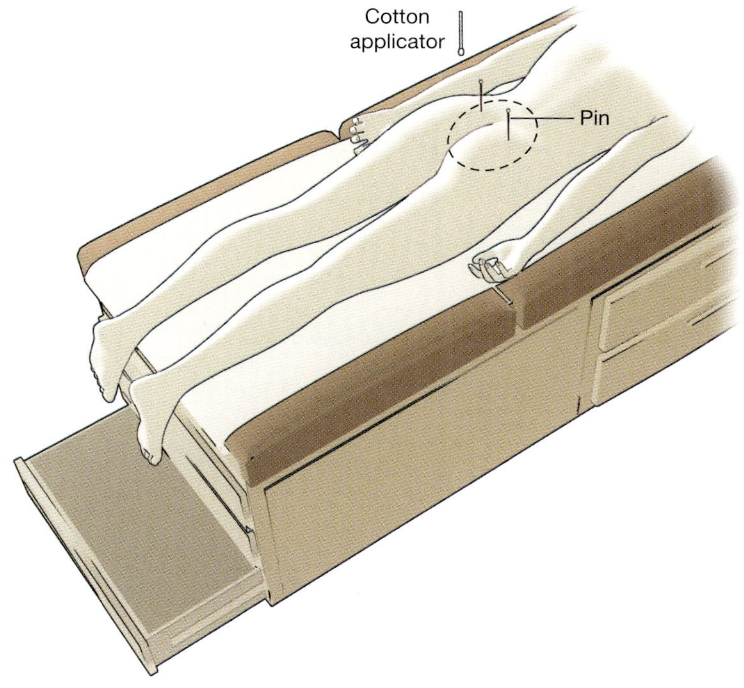

FIGURE 3-16: Testing for Saddle Anesthesia

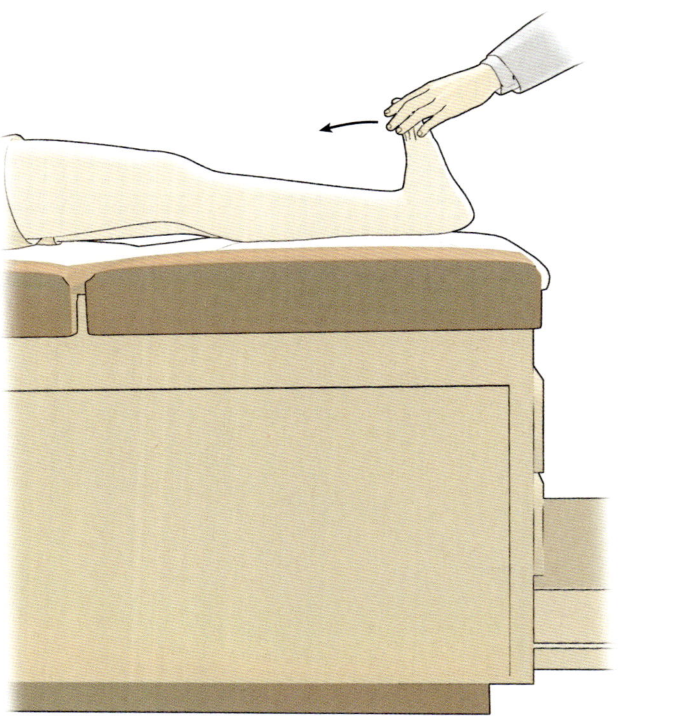

FIGURE 3-17: Power Dorsiflexion of Foot and Toes

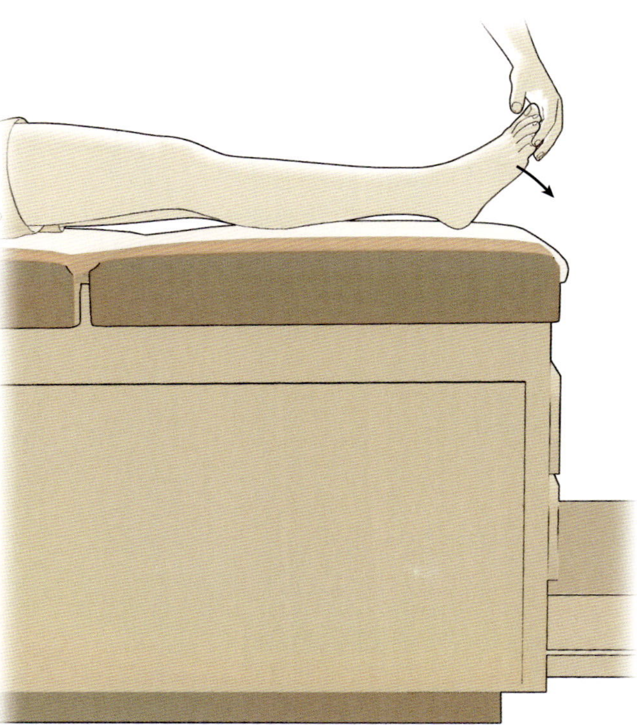

FIGURE 3-18: Power Plantar Flexion of Foot and Toes

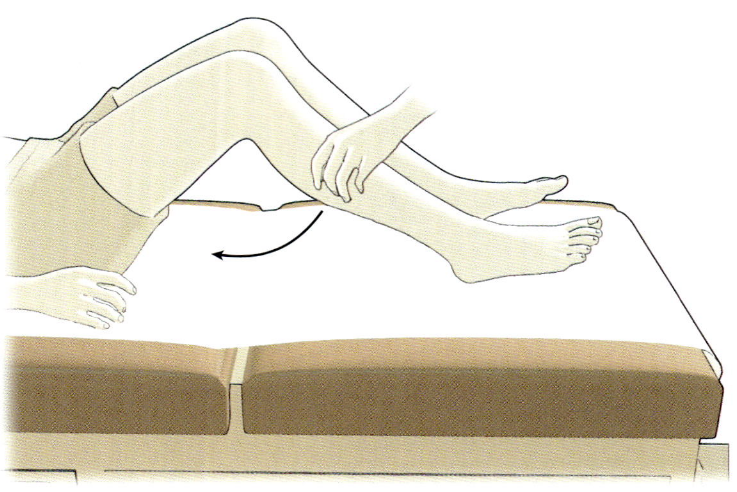

FIGURE 3-19: Power Flexion at the Knee

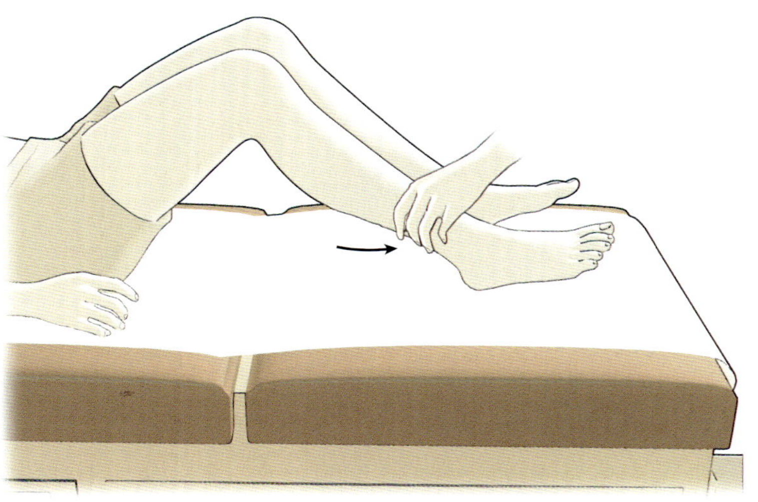

FIGURE 3-20: Power Extension at the Knee

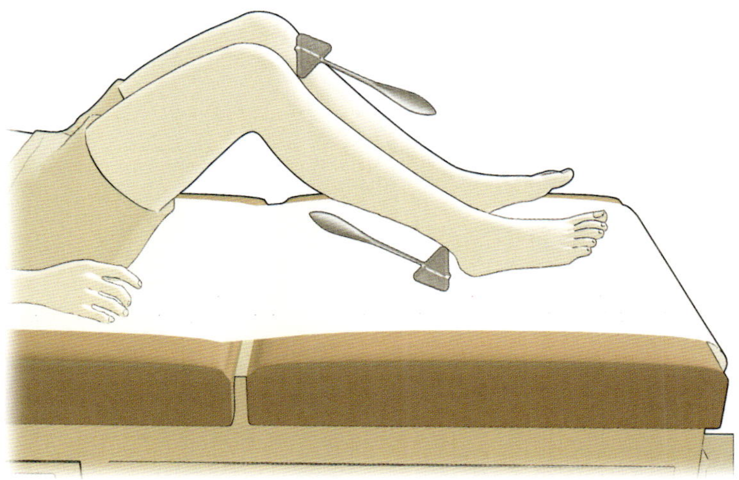

FIGURE 3-21: Reflexes Knee Jerk and Ankle Jerk

Look for atrophy (usually a clear indication for surgery) at the calf and thigh by measuring the circumference of the calf at the bulkiest point on each leg and the circumference of the thigh at just above the knee (Figure 3-22). Compare the results on one leg with the other.

Look for fasciculations of the muscles of the thigh and calf if you have not already observed for them before (Figure 3-23). The possibility that the back and/or hip pain are due to hip pathology always exists, so perform a Patrick test (Figure 3-24) by crossing each lower leg over the opposite thigh and pressing the knee of the crossed leg to see if pain can be elicited. If pain is elicited, check further for hip pathology. Finally, palpate the back for trigger points and sacroiliac tenderness (Figure 3-25). Check for malingering or hysteria by doing an axial rotation test (Figure 3-26). With the patient standing and one hand on the shoulder and the other on the opposite hip, rotate the patient's body to the right and left. If back pain is elicited, the patient is likely malingering. Be sure to check the arterial pulses (Figure 3-27) to be sure the leg pain is not vascular in origin. Table 3-2 summarizes the neurologic findings in the most common forms of lumbar radiculopathy.

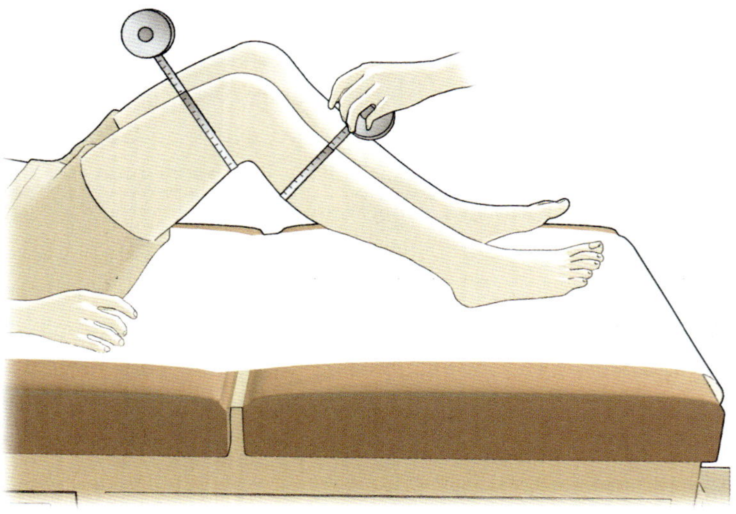

FIGURE 3-22: Measure Calf and Thigh

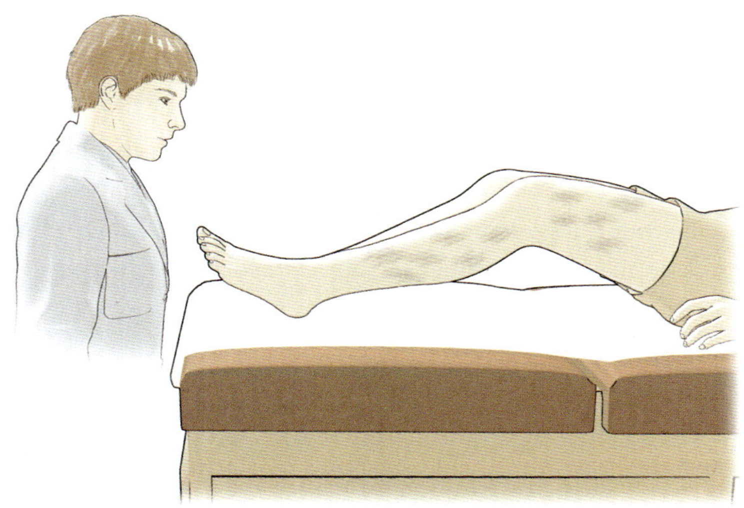

FIGURE 3-23: Look for Fasciculations

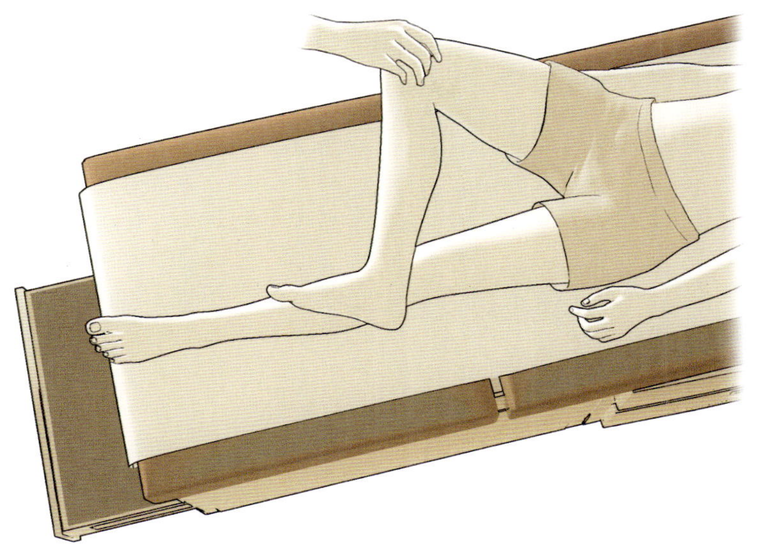

FIGURE 3-24: Patrick Test Hip Pathology

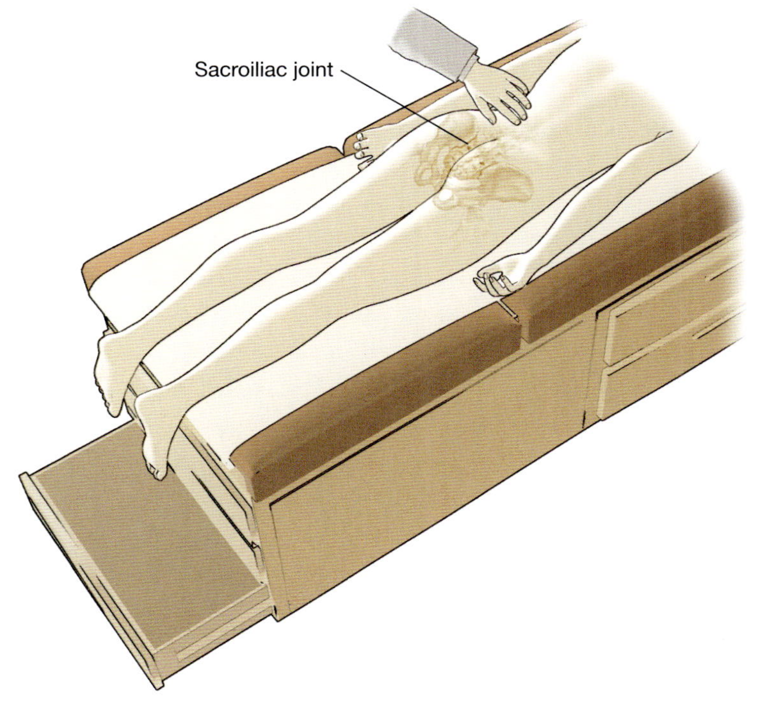

FIGURE 3-25: Palpate for Trigger Points and Sacroiliac Tenderness

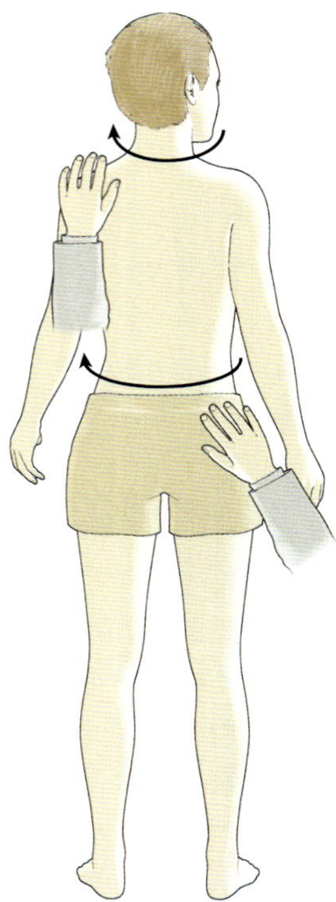

FIGURE 3-26: Axial Rotation Test

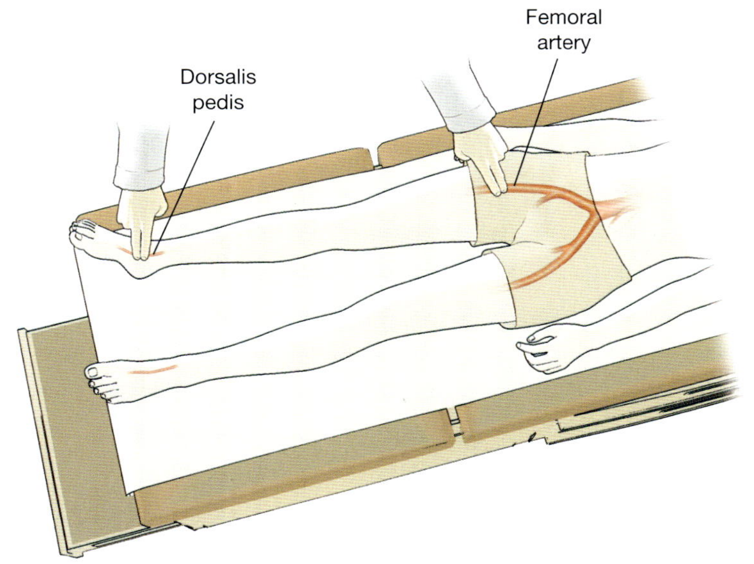

FIGURE 3-27: Examine Arterial Pulses

TABLE 3-2

Neurologic Findings in the Most Common Forms of Lumbar Radiculopathy

Nerve Root Involved	Weakness	Loss of Sensation	Loss of Reflexes
L4	Quadriceps	Anterior thigh and knee Medial lower leg	Knee jerk
L5	Dorsi-flexion of big toe	Dorsum of foot and big toe	None
S1	Flexion of toes and extension of foot	Lateral foot and little toe	Ankle jerk

C Diagnosis of the Patient with Low Back Pain

After the completion of the history and physical examination, you may have a reasonably good idea of what you are dealing with but deciding how to proceed with the workup at this point may be confusing. There's a way to alleviate any indecisiveness. Basically, you will be presented with four scenarios.

1. **Low back pain without radiation, with a history of trauma but no evidence of radiculopathy.** The diagnosis here is either a lumbosacral sprain or in rare cases a fracture. Plain films to screen for a fracture would be indicated, but ordering laboratory or other diagnostic tests may be unnecessary unless the patient fails to respond to conservative therapy. A CT scan may be necessary to show a fracture in some cases.
2. **Low back pain without radiation, without a history of trauma and with no evidence of radiculopathy.** These patients probably have a lumbosacral sprain or spondylosis and can be treated conservatively. However, if you haven't already done so, perform a thorough abdominal examination to exclude an abdominal aneurysm, and other conditions. Perform a rectal examination in males to look for prostatitis and prostatic carcinoma, and a pelvic examination to look for PID, endometriosis, and uterine or ovarian tumors in females. A CBC, sedimentation rate, chemistry and

arthritis panel, and a PSA may also be helpful. Young males should be tested for HLA-B27 antigen. Plain films of the lumbosacral spine would seem indicated, but some authorities feel these are unnecessary unless the patient fails to respond to conservative therapy.[1]

3. **Low back pain with or without a history of trauma with evidence of radiculopathy, but without significant weakness in the lower extremities, and no atrophy or loss of bladder control.** These patients can also be treated conservatively, but plain films of the lumbosacral spine, CBC, sedimentation rate, chemistry, and arthritis panel would be indicated. These patients most likely have a herniated disc, spinal stenosis, or spondylosis with foraminal encroachment on one or more lumbosacral nerve roots. In females, they may also have a pelvic tumor or endometriosis. When these patients fail to respond to conservative treatment, a referral to a neurologist or neurosurgeon is clearly indicated before ordering expensive diagnostic tests such as an MRI, CT, or bone scan. An NCV and EMG study of the lower extremity will help differentiate radiculopathy from a neuropathy.[2]
4. **Low back pain with or without a history of trauma, with definite evidence of radiculopathy** or obvious lower extremity weakness (such as a footdrop), atrophy of the thighs or calves, or a cauda equina syndrome as evidenced by loss of bladder and/or rectal control, erectile dysfunction, or saddle anesthesia. These cases would require immediate referral to a neurosurgeon. It is not the place of a primary care provider to order MRIs, CT scans, or other expensive diagnostic tests when there is such an obvious indication for surgery in these cases.[1]

D Conservative Management of the Patient with Low Back Pain

The various treatment options for low back pain are listed in Table 3-3.

Acute Low Back Pain: As is the case with acute neck and thoracic pain, once you have ruled out an abdominal or pelvic condition the mainstay of therapy is nonnarcotic *analgesics* (acetaminophen, etc.), *NSAIDs* such as

TABLE 3-3

Conservative Management of Low Back Pain

1. Analgesics
2. Nonsteroidal anti-inflammatory Drugs
3. Muscle relaxants
4. Corticosteroids
5. Reducing diet
6. Lumbar support
7. Physiotherapy
8. Exercise
9. Heel and sole inserts
10. Trigger point Injections
11. Facet injections
12. Epidural corticosteroids
13. Antidepressants
14. Anticonvulsants
15. Prayer

ibuprofen 600 to 800 mg T.I.D. or naproxen 250 to 500 mg B.I.D. and *muscle relaxants* such as cyclobenzaprine (Flexeril) 10 mg T.I.D. or metaxalone (Skelaxin) 800 mg T.I.D. It is questionable whether muscle relaxants other than carisoprodol (Soma) or the benzodiazepines (diazepam, etc.) are effective but the latter are habit forming, which limits their use. Short courses of *narcotics* such as APAP with codeine or hydrocodone (Vicodin) may be prescribed. If the pain seems unbearable, perhaps hospitalization for parenteral narcotics would be advisable.

A short course of *corticosteroids* (Medrol Dosepak or prednisone 30 mg daily and tapering over 7 to 10 days) may be therapeutic. As suggested above, alternate-day steroids may be successful. The author has also used intramuscular corticosteroids such as triamcinolone acetonide (Kenalog) on many occasions with good results especially when combined with oral NSAIDs. These injections should not be administered more frequently than every 2 weeks.

Lumbar supports are also useful because they limit ROM and really do provide stabilization of the lumbar spine for this reason: A hollow tube is stronger than a solid tube (basic physics). And the immediate strengthening of the ABS creates the "hollow tube." Trigger point, sacroiliac and facet injections with lidocaine 1% to 2% may also be tried. Sometimes combining this with a corticosteroid gives more lasting relief. The author hesitates to start these patients on physiotherapy because this can become addicting especially if there is litigation pending.

Chronic Low Back Pain: Once again a patient presenting with long-standing low back pain (more than 12 weeks) can be managed with nonnarcotic analgesics, NSAIDs and muscle relaxants. If these have already been utilized, try a different NSAID such as meloxicam, celecoxib (Celebrex) or diclofenac (Voltaren). Beyond that, try a different muscle relaxant. Caution: Prescribing narcotics for chronic low back pain is forbidden. Alternate-day steroids as described above have been successful in many cases.

If there is inequality of leg length, order a heel and sole insert for the short leg.

Alternatively, have a shoemaker build up the heel and sole of the shoe on the short leg on all shoes worn frequently. Get rid of flip-flops for the time being.

Obese patients absolutely must be put on a *reducing diet* like the fruit and vegetable diet mentioned under neck pain (Table 1-4). This is especially important if surgery is anticipated later. Lumbar supports especially to be worn at night are also useful. These are also helpful to patients whose jobs require long periods of sitting.

Don't let the patient with chronic low back pain leave the office without an exercise program. Table 3-4, which details the use of sit-ups and pelvic tilts, is the best in the author's opinion.[3] The technique for performing these exercises is illustrated in Figure 3-28.

Physiotherapy is another option, but let the physiotherapist or a physiatrist decide on the form of treatment. Remember that this can become addicting especially if there is pending litigation.

"Chiropractic manipulation is no more effective than a popular form of physiotherapy" according to Cherkin et al.[4]

Trigger point, facet, and sacroiliac injections with 1% to 2% lidocaine are often worthwhile especially when combined with corticosteroids (10 to

TABLE 3-4

Exercises for the Patient with Low Back Pain

Purpose—To strengthen the anterior spinal muscles (psoas major, etc.) and anterior abdominal muscles (rectus abdominis, etc.)

1. Pelvic tilts
   a. Lie down on a solid surface with legs flexed at the knees.
   b. Place one hand underneath the lumbar spine.
   c. Tilt pelvis backwards, pressing the lumbar spine against the hand, and count to 10 slowly.
   d. Relax and repeat.
   e. Begin performing this 10 minutes twice a day until you reach 30 minutes twice a day. Some patients benefit by increasing to 30 minutes three times a day.
2. Sit-ups
   a. Lie down on a solid surface with legs extended and anchored by a couch or another person holding the feet.
   b. With arms extended at a 90-degree angle with your body, sit up slowly and touch your knees.
   c. Return to the recumbent position slowly and relax.
   d. Repeat this procedure 10 times twice a day gradually increasing to 50 times twice a day over a period of 4–6 weeks. Maintain the integrity of your anterior spinal muscles and ABS by performing this exercise three times a week indefinitely.

40 mg of triamcinolone acetonide [Kenalog]). There is no need to penetrate the facet joint when giving the injections. Getting the needle close to the joint will suffice. If the primary care provider is uncomfortable performing these procedures, he/she should not hesitate to refer the patient to an orthopedic or neurologic specialist or someone experienced in these techniques.

The same applies to epidural corticosteroid injections. However, administering these by the caudal approach is certainly feasible for the primary care provider if he or she will follow the steps outlined in Table 3-5 adapted from my article published in the Journal of Neurological and Orthopedic Medicine and Surgery.[5] Figure 3-29 illustrates the technique for performing an epidural by the caudal approach.

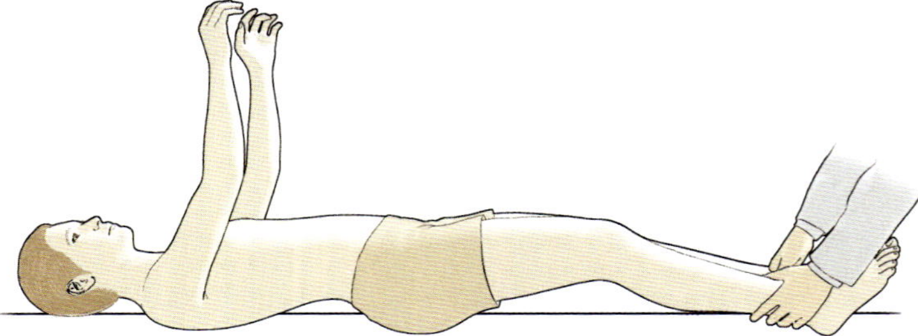

1. Patient lies flat, legs and arms extended, someone holding legs down.

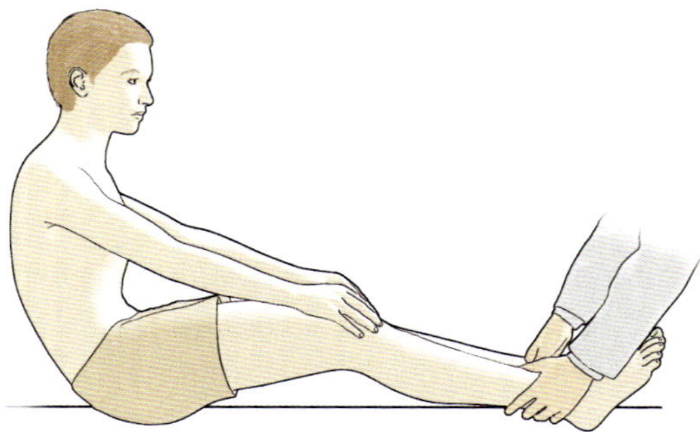

2. Patient sits up, touching knees, no further. Repeat steps 1 and 2 10–50 times beginning with 10 and gradually increasing by 5 a week.

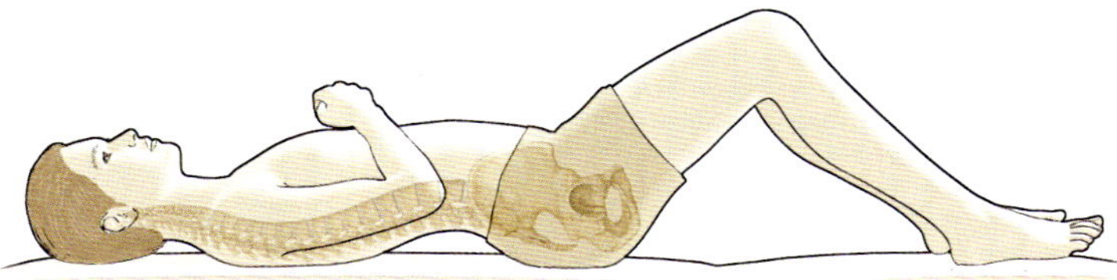

1. Lumbar spine is arched, knees flexed.

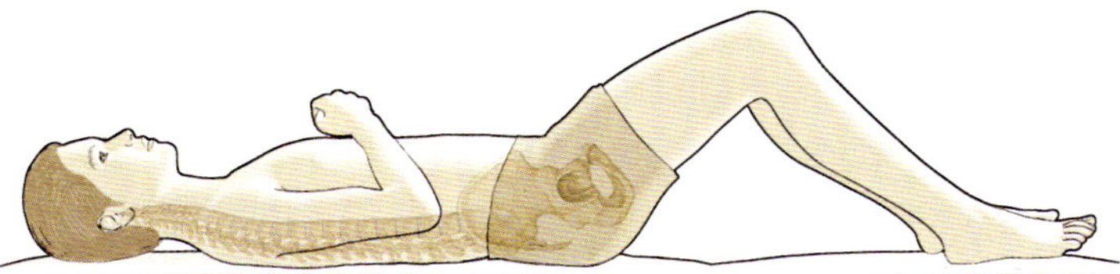

2. Lumbar spine is flattened against surface, pelvis rotates posteriorly.

FIGURE 3-28: Exercises for the Patient with Low Back Pain

TABLE 3-5

Technique of Performing an Epidural Injection by the Caudal Approach

1. The patient's sacral area is prepped with 10% povidone–iodine solution (Betadine) and draped appropriately.
2. Locate the sacral hiatus between the prominent sacral cornu and mark with a nail impression.
3. Draw 8 cc of 1.5% lidocaine (for caudal use) and 2 cc (80 mg) of triamcinolone acetonide (Kenalog) into a 10 cc syringe with a 1.5-inches, 22-gauge needle.
4. Put on a pair of sterile gloves and again located the sacral hiatus. Prep the area again.
5. Insert the needle into the hiatus at a 60-degree angle for ½ to 1 and ½ inches or until resistance is encountered.
6. Then withdraw the needle slightly and angle it a bit more rostrally for another quarter to one-half inch.
7. The barrel of the syringe is withdrawn slightly with gentle pressure to be sure the needle is not in a vein, and then the contents of the syringe are injected slowly 2 cc at a time. This is to be sure that a bolus of the contents is not injected into a vein as this may cause respiratory arrest (a rare complication).
8. A moderate amount of resistance may be encountered, but if there is too little or too much, you should withdraw the needle and reposition it again.
9. After the injection, place a small Band-Aid at the sight of the patient's injection and monitor pulse and respiration for 10 min before releasing the patient to the waiting room.
10. I insist they remain in the waiting room or recovery room for another half hour and have someone drive them home.

Adapted from Collins RD. One hundred consecutive epidural injections for back pain. *J Neurol Orthop Med Surg.* 1991;12:120–123, with permission.

A couple of words of caution are indicated:

1. Make sure the patient has never had a reaction to lidocaine before.
2. Inject the solution slowly, observing for suppressed respirations in case the needle is in a vein.
3. Try a normal saline injection first to gain some experience with the procedure.

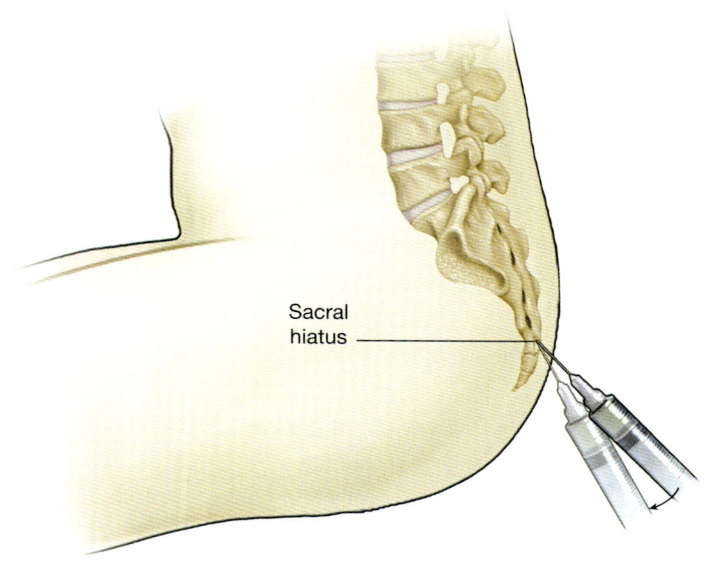

FIGURE 3-29: Epidural Injection by the Caudal Approach

(You may be pleasantly surprised to find that normal saline works!)

Be sure to warn the patient about complications such as a cauda equina hematoma or epidural abscess. The author instructs his patients to go immediately to the emergency room if there is anything peculiar happening in the few days following the procedure and routinely calls the patient within 24 hours of the injection just to be sure there are no complications.

Antidepressants such as duloxetine (Cymbalta) 40 to 60 mg B.I.D. and anticonvulsants such as gabapentin (Neurontin) 300 to 800 mg T.I.D. may be prescribed but are best left for the pain management specialist to administer.

Surgical options are listed in Table 3-6. It is not in the scope of this textbook to discuss which procedure should be used in any individual case, as this is up to the experience and expertise of the neurosurgeon or orthopedic specialist.

Figure 3-30 depicts an algorithm of the management of low back pain that should help the primary care provider in his or her decision-making.

TABLE 3-6

Surgical Management of Low Back Pain

1. Laminectomy/discectomy
2. Microdiscectomy/microendoscopic approach
3. Posterolateral, posterior lumbar interbody fusion
4. Transforaminal interbody fusion
5. Anterior lumbar interbody fusion

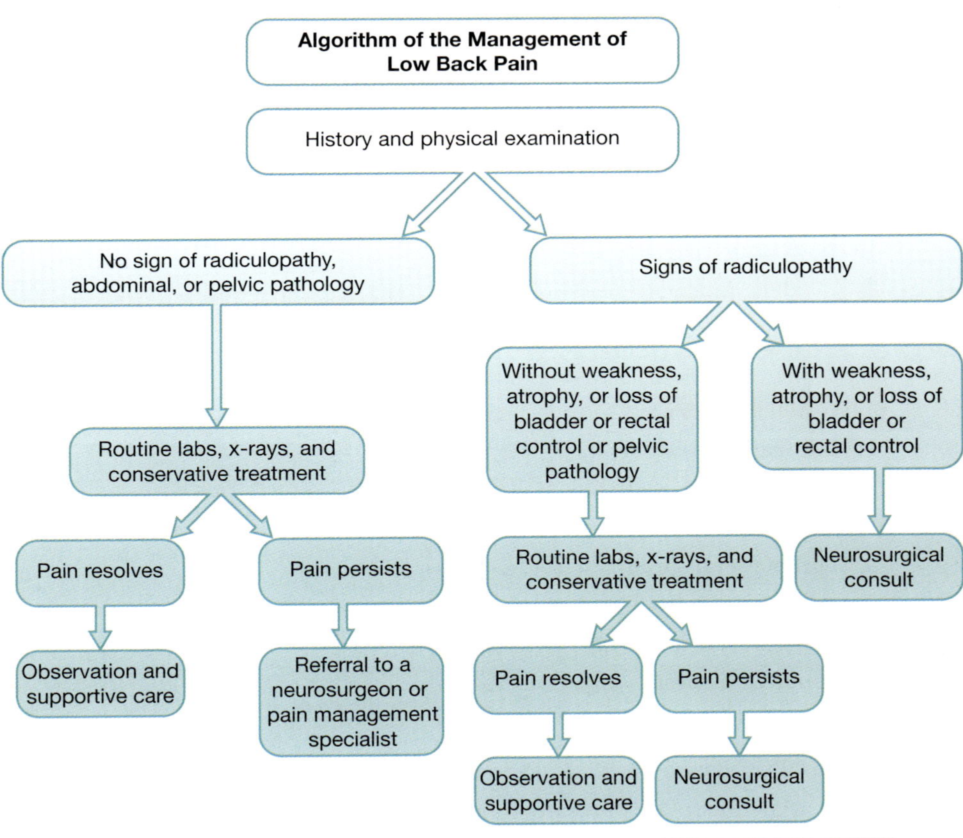

FIGURE 3-30: Algorithm of the Management of Low Back Pain

E Illustrated Cases of Low Back Pain

Normal Anatomy of the Lumbosacral Spine (Figure 3-31)

Herniated Disc L5-S1 (Figure 3-32)

A 46-year-old nurse complained of acute onset of low back pain radiating down the left leg after turning a patient over in his bed. The pain increased on coughing and almost any activity.

Physical examination revealed a positive SLR at 40 degrees on the left, limited ROM of the lumbar spine, absent left Achilles reflex, and diminished sensation to touch and pain on the lateral foot and little toe.

Plain films of the lumbar spine were unremarkable, but an MRI revealed a large disc herniation at L5-S1 on the left.

Conservative Treatment was unsuccessful. The patient recovered after a hemilaminectomy.

Differential Diagnosis

1. Lumbar spondylosis
2. Osteoarthritis of the hip
3. Sacroiliitis
4. Lumbosacral sprain
5. Pelvic pathology
6. Scoliosis due to short leg syndrome
7. Spondylolisthesis

Discussion: This case is typical of a traumatic induced herniated disc. Some would argue that plain films are unnecessary to rule out other pathology. It is always prudent to try conservative treatment before surgery in these cases because a laminectomy is only 70% to 80% successful and while relieving the radiculopathy, there may be continuous low back pain for years following surgery in some cases.

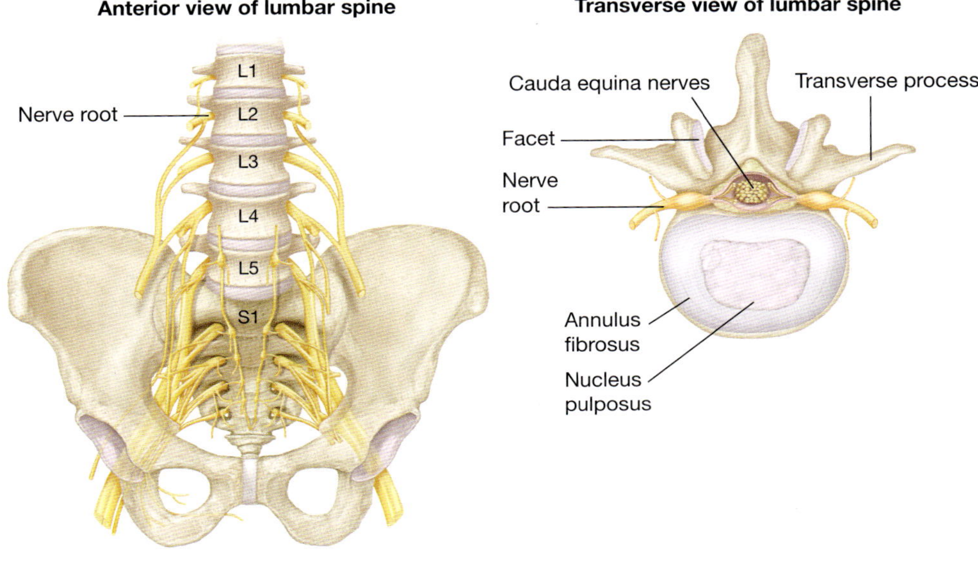

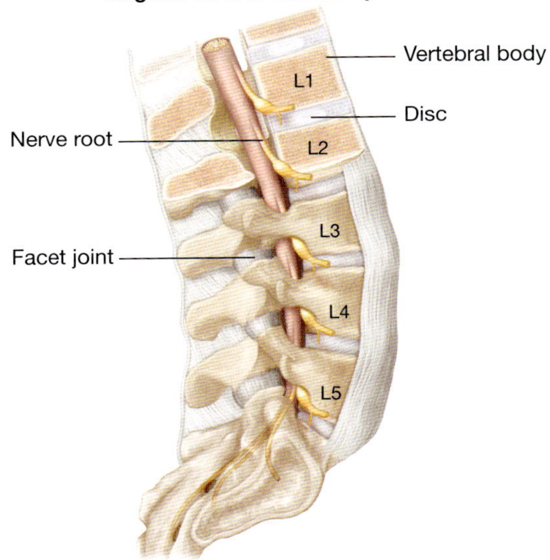

FIGURE 3-31: Normal Anatomy of the Lumbosacral Spine

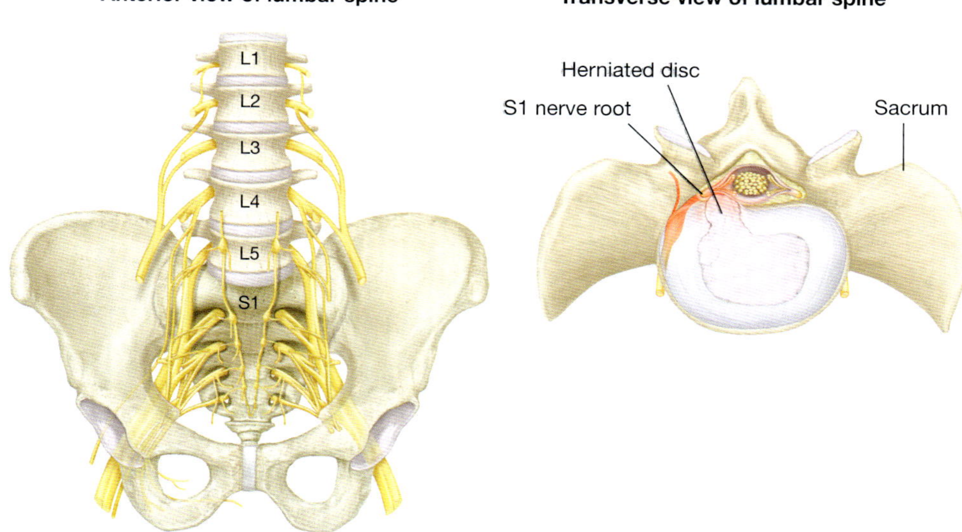

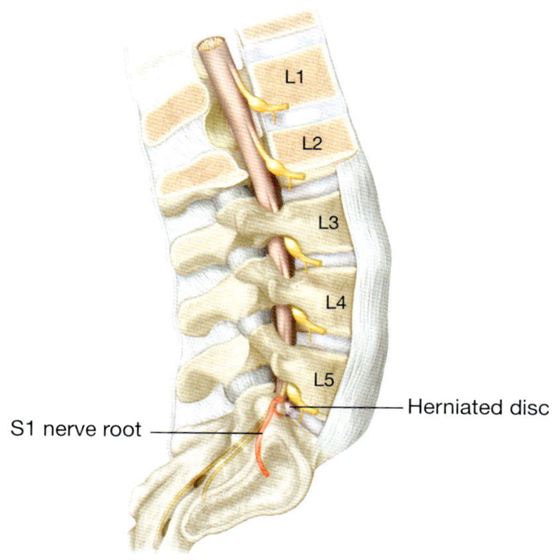

FIGURE 3-32: Herniated Disc (L5-S1)

Herniated Disc L3-L4 (Figure 3-33)

A 38-year-old truck driver presented to the ER with acute low back pain radiating into his right thigh that began while unloading his truck.

Past History revealed he had already had surgery for a herniated disc of the spine with good results 3 years previously.

Neurologic examination revealed severe bilateral erector spine muscle spasm, weakness on extension of his right leg at the knee, diminished sensation to touch and pain over the right knee and medial surface of the tibia, as well as a loss of his patellar reflex. Femoral stretch test was positive on the right at 45 degrees.

Routine laboratory studies were unremarkable, but plain films of the lumbar spine showed degenerative changes as well as narrowing of the disc spaces at L3-L4 and L5-S1.

Treatment: His primary care provider treated him with bed rest, NSAIDs, and muscle relaxants. When after 6 weeks he failed to show improvement, he was referred to a neurosurgeon.

Differential Diagnosis

1. Lumbar spondylosis
2. Primary or metastatic neoplasm
3. Epidural abscess
4. Lumbosacral sprain
5. Compression fracture
6. Spondylolisthesis

Discussion: Notice that an MRI was not ordered by the primary care provider. This is the most cost-effective approach to the management of disorders of the lumbosacral spine.[6] With positive findings on the neurologic examination, a neurologic consult would have been wise, however.

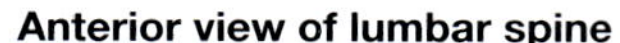

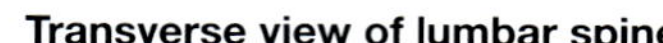

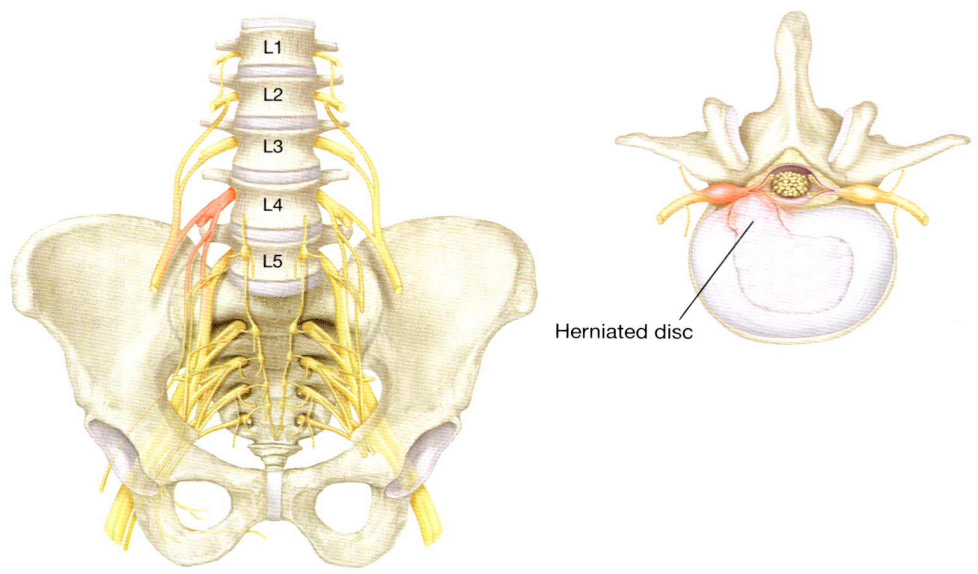

Sagittal view of lumbar spine

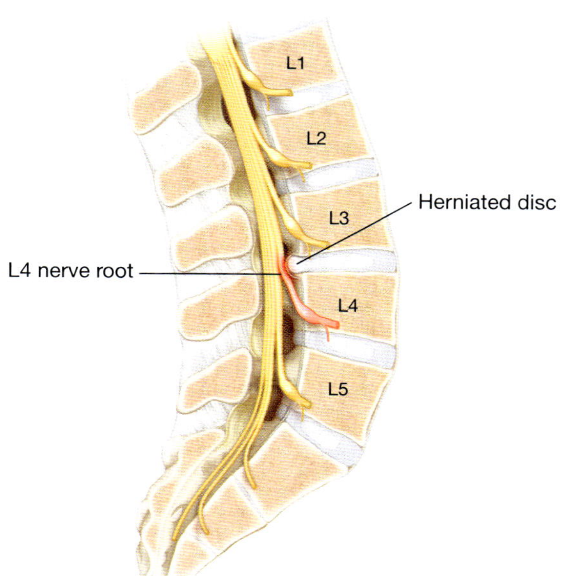

FIGURE 3-33: Herniated Disc (L3-L4)

Metastatic Carcinoma of the Lumbar Spine (Figure 3-34)

A 67-year-old black male complained of increasing low back pain for the past 6 months with radiation into both lower extremities in the past 6 weeks. He presented to the ER with incontinence of urine and feces for the past week.

Neurologic examination revealed a short step gait, absent Achilles reflexes bilaterally, weakness of flexion of the feet and toes bilaterally, and diminished sensation on the lateral aspect of his lower legs and feet. A rectal examination reveals an enlarged nodular prostate with loss of sphincter tone and control.

Laboratory studies revealed a marked elevation of his PSA and acid and alkaline phosphatases.

X-rays of the lumbosacral spine showed diffuse erosive lesions worse at L5-S1 with degenerative disease consistent with his age.

Treatment: Immediate neurosurgical and urologic referral was made, but radiation and androgen-deprivation therapy allowed only partial relief of his pain and no improvement in his disability.

Differential Diagnosis

1. Epidural abscess
2. Large herniated disc
3. Rectal carcinoma with metastasis.
4. Multiple myeloma
5. Lumbar spondylosis with spinal stenosis

Discussion: This is a typical case of cauda equina syndrome, which must be referred to a neurosurgeon immediately if there is any hope for a resolution.

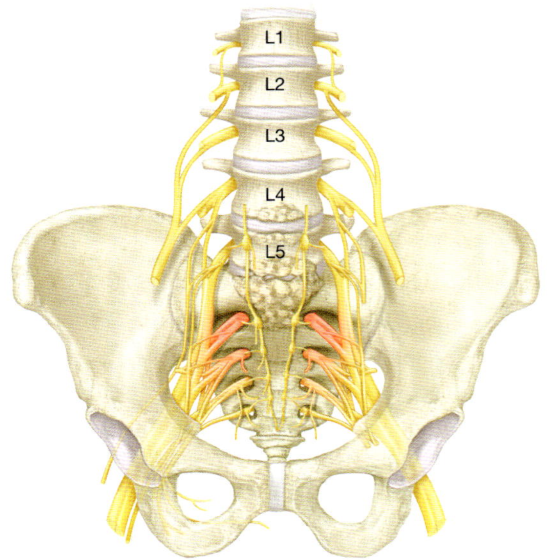

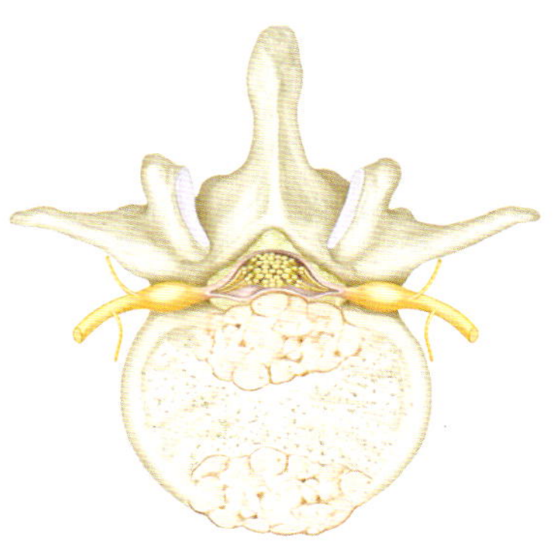

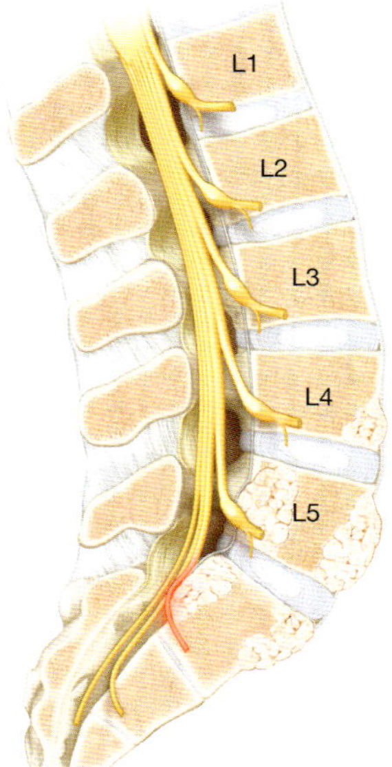

FIGURE 3-34: Metastatic Carcinoma

Spondylolisthesis (Figure 3-35)

A 42-year-old obese female complained of increasing low back pain for 3 years. In the past 6 months, she has noticed pain, numbness, and tingling of both lower extremities. Prolonged standing and walking caused increasing pain in her buttocks and thighs (neurogenic claudication).

Neurologic examination revealed weakness of extension of both big toes, loss of sensation on the dorsum of the feet and big toes, and a pelvic tilt.

Plain films demonstrated the anterior slippage of the 5th lumbar vertebrae on the sacrum and the typical "scotty dog" appearance of the pars interarticularis.

Treatment: The patient failed to respond to conservative treatment with NSAIDs and a lumbosacral support but improved following reduction and posterolateral fusion.

Differential Diagnosis

1. Herniated disc
2. Cauda equina tumor
3. Epidural abscess
4. Leriche syndrome
5. Ovarian cyst
6. Lumbar spondylosis
7. Scoliosis

Discussion: Unless there is a high degree of slippage, most of these cases respond to conservative treatment. An MRI is useful to show the stenosis of the foramina but is not necessary unless surgery is contemplated. As in all cases of low back pain that do not respond to conservative treatment, a referral to a neurosurgeon is indicated before ordering an MRI or other expensive diagnostic tests.

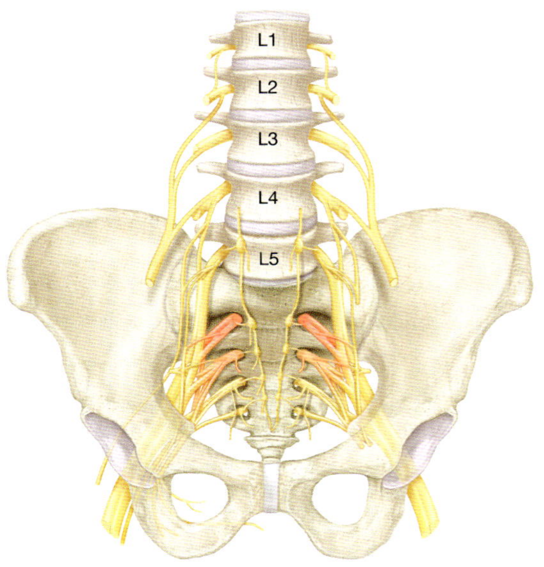

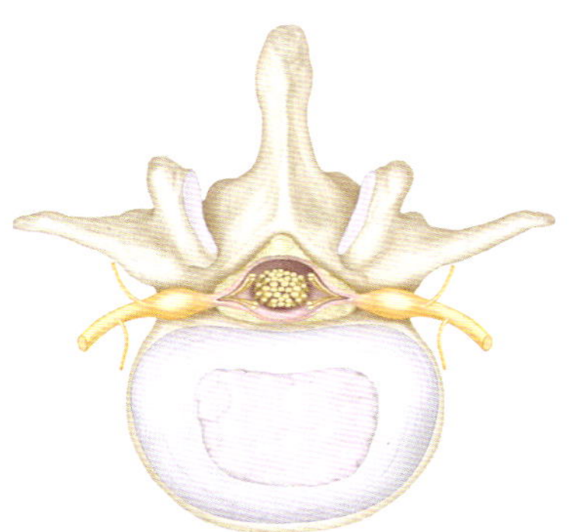

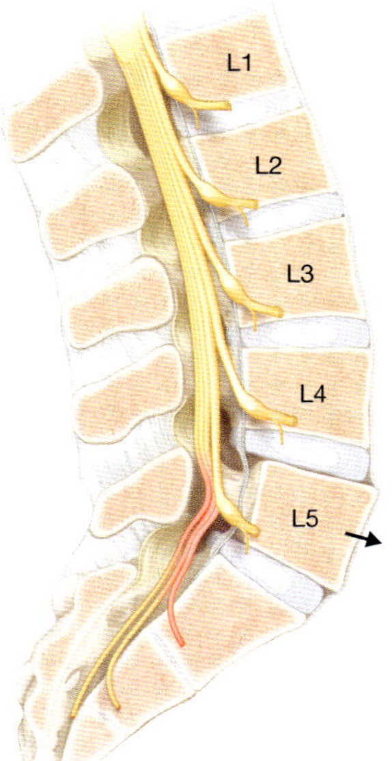

FIGURE 3-35: Spondylolisthesis

Lumbar Spondylosis with Spinal Stenosis (Figure 3-36)

An 80-year-old physician complained of twitching and cramps in his lower extremities for several months. On further questioning, he stated he had had low back pain for many years and numbness and tingling in both lower extremities for at least 4 years.

Review of systems revealed he also had erectile dysfunction and difficulty voiding for at least 2 years.

Past history was negative for diabetes or alcoholism but disclosed an episode of severe low back pain following lifting a heavy organ 30 years ago.

Neurologic examination showed fasciculations of calves and tibialis anterior muscles but no other objective findings.

A plain films of his lumbar spine showed marked narrowing of his L5-S1 disc space and degenerative changes at L3-L4, L4-L5, and L5-S1.

An MRI was diagnostic of severe central spinal canal stenosis with severe bilateral facet arthropathy at L3-L4, L4-L5, and L5-S1, as well as a 6- to 7-mm diffuse bulging of the disc at L3-L4.

Treatment: While surgery was recommended, the patient elected to have conservative treatment with inversion, exercises, NSAIDs, and epidural steroid injections. Two years later, he has not changed his mind.

Differential Diagnosis

1. Herniated disc
2. Primary or metastatic neoplasm
3. Peripheral or aortic arteriosclerosis
4. Multiple myeloma
5. Epidural abscess
6. Spondylolisthesis

Discussion: Sadly, many patients with a herniated disc or severe spinal stenosis will elect conservative treatment over surgery because of mixed results in at least 20% of cases. Relief of radiculopathy is almost certain, but the low back pain continues in many cases.

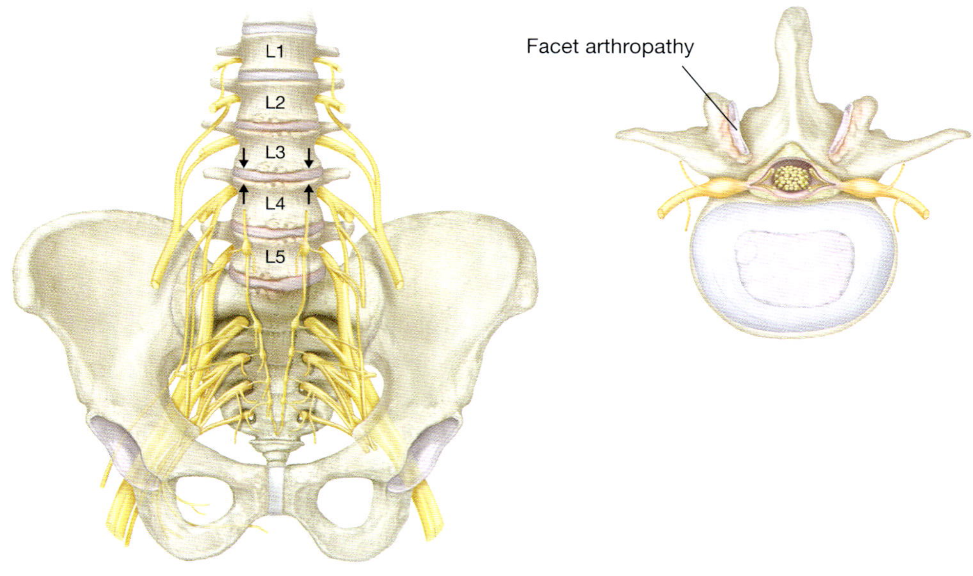

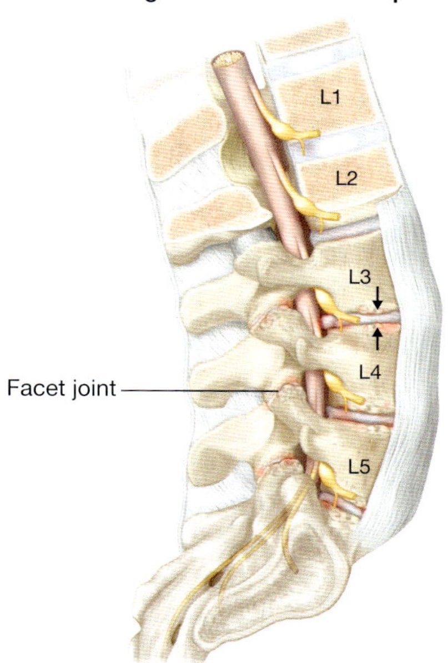

FIGURE 3-36: Lumbar Spondylosis with Spinal Stenosis

Leriche Syndrome: Arteriosclerosis of the Aorta and Femoral Arteries (Figure 3-37)

A 54-year-old white male complained of increasing numbness and tingling in both legs for several months associated with exquisite cramps in both legs on walking one block (intermittent claudication). Because of MRI findings of lumbar spondylosis he was admitted to the neurosurgical service for possible laminectomy and fusion. He was a heavy smoker.

Neurologic examination showed absent deep tendon reflexes and distal hypesthesia and hypalgesia in both lower extremities, but no pathologic reflexes. Femoral, popliteal, dorsalis pedis, and tibialis pulses were barely palpable bilaterally, and there were bruits over both femoral arteries.

Routine x-rays of the abdomen and pelvis showed calcification of the terminal aorta and femoral arteries, and severe arteriosclerosis of the terminal aorta and femoral arteries was confirmed on angiography.

Differential Diagnosis

1. Spinal stenosis
2. Aortic aneurysm with dissection
3. Pelvic tumor
4. Metastatic carcinoma of the spine
5. Epidural abscess
6. Peripheral neuropathy
7. Herniated disc

Treatment: Endarterectomy was successful in relieving the patient's symptoms.

Discussion: This patient emphasizes that clinicians must examine the peripheral pulses in patients presenting with neurologic symptoms of the lower extremities or low back pain especially when there is increasing pain on ambulation (neurogenic vs. vascular intermittent claudication).

Anterior view of lumbar spine

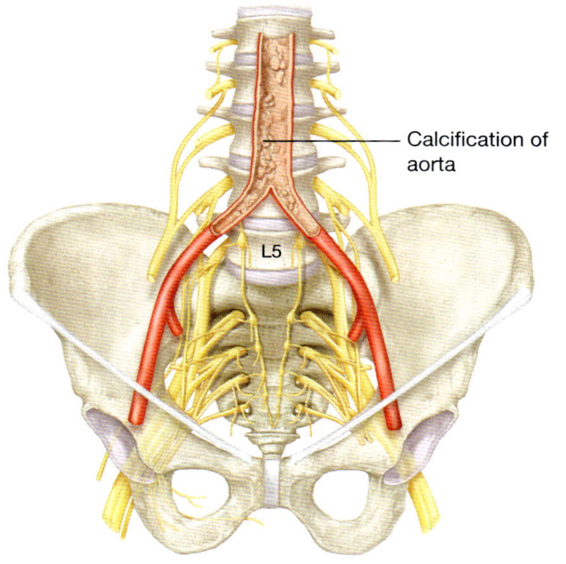

Transverse view of lumbar spine

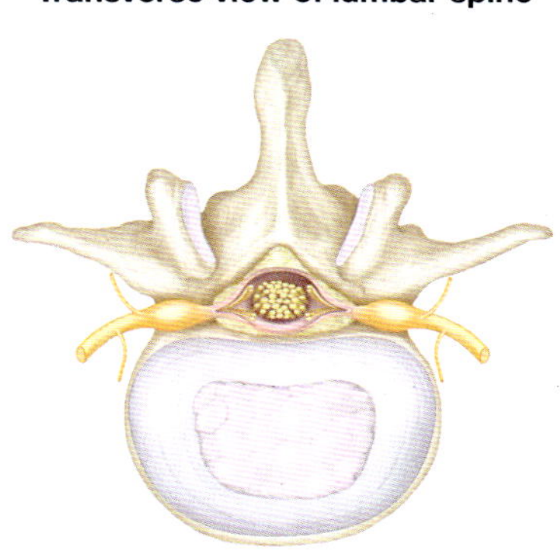

Sagittal view of lumbar spine

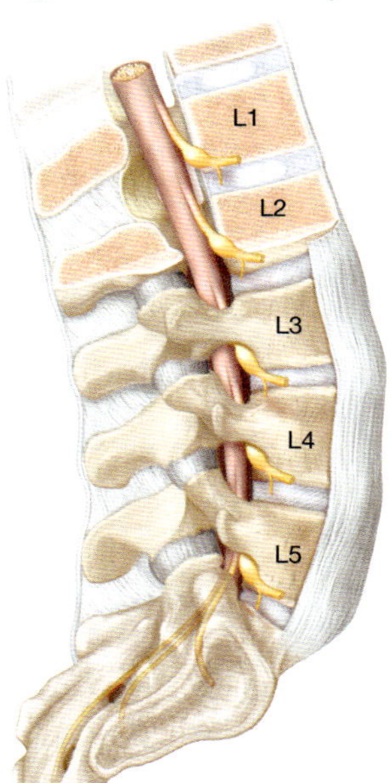

FIGURE 3-37: Leriche Syndrome (Atherosclerosis of the Terminal Aorta)

Ovarian Cyst (Figure 3-38)

A 48-year-old white female was being treated successfully for low back pain supposedly due to lumbar spondylosis with epidural corticosteroids by an anesthesiologist. However, following her last injection 3 months prior to admission, she developed increasing low back pain radiating to her left extremity, associated with mild weakness, numbness, and tingling in both lower extremities. These symptoms were blamed on her last epidural, and she saw a lawyer with the intention of filing a suit against the anesthesiologist.

Neurologic examination by an independent medical examiner failed to show any objective findings, and a repeat MRI of the lumbar spine interpreted by her local radiologist failed to show anything other than the degenerative changes found on previous MRIs.

Upon *review of the MRIs* by a second radiologist, a large ovarian cyst was found.

Treatment: A large ovarian cystadenoma was removed at surgery, and the patient's symptoms resolved postoperatively.

Differential Diagnosis

1. Lumbar spondylosis
2. Herniated lumbar disc
3. Cauda equina syndrome
4. Osteoporosis
5. Aortic aneurysm
6. Epidural abscess
7. Endometriosis
8. Pelvic inflammatory disease

Discussion: This case emphasizes that abdominal and pelvic disorders must be looked for when patients fail to respond to conventional therapy.[7]

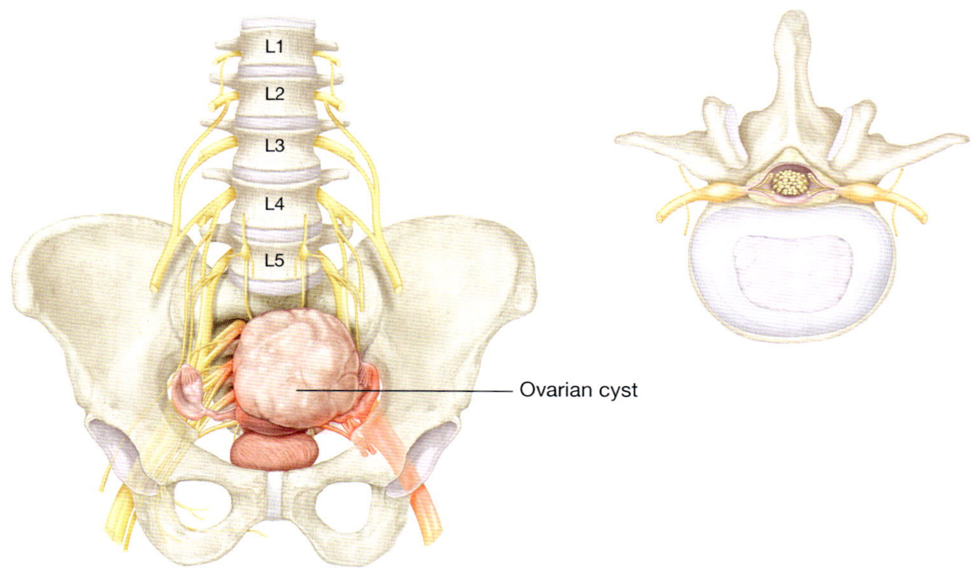

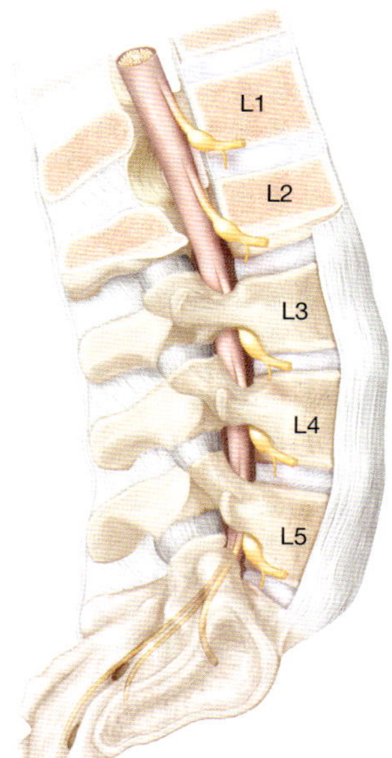

FIGURE 3-38: Ovarian Cyst

Scoliosis due to a Short Leg Syndrome (Figure 3-39)

A 53-year-old white male, owner of a snowmobile rental company, complained of long-standing low back pain that occasionally radiated down his left leg. There was no increase of the pain on coughing and sneezing and no history of injury. Years ago, he was told he had scoliosis by a chiropractor.

Physical examination revealed moderate tenderness and spasm of the erector spinae muscles worse on the left, but sensation, power, and reflexes were intact in the lower extremities, and SLR and femoral stretch tests were negative. However, his right leg was 1 inch shorter than the left. x-Rays of the lumbosacral spine including an AP standing view revealed scoliosis convex to the right.

Laboratory examination was unremarkable.

Treatment: A ½ inch heel and sole insert in the right shoe resulted in total relief of his pain within 1 week.

Differential Diagnosis

1. Lumbosacral sprain
2. Lumbar spondylosis
3. Idiopathic scoliosis
4. Herniated lumbar disc
5. Rheumatoid spondylitis

Discussion: Twenty percent of patients with chronic low back pain have scoliosis due to a significant shortening of one leg in the author's experience. These patients uniformly respond to an insert in the shoe of the affected leg. Alternatively a shoemaker can build up the heel and sole on all shoes worn frequently.

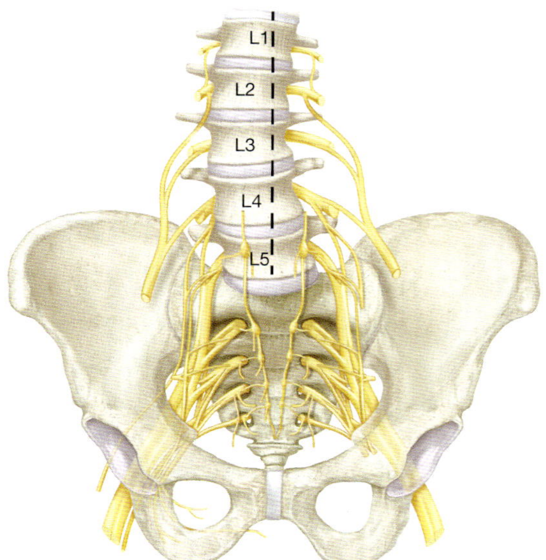

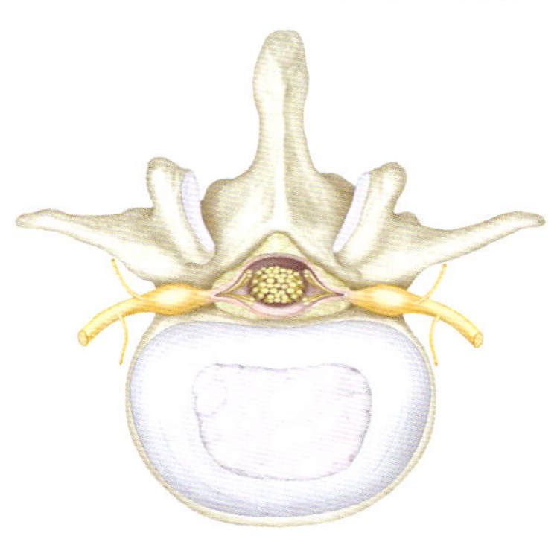

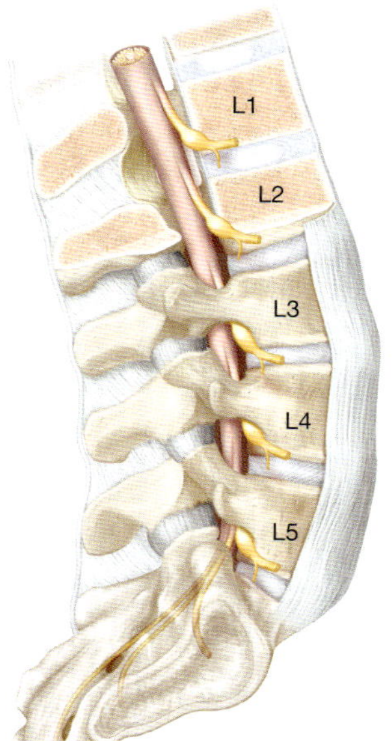

FIGURE 3-39: Scoliosis Due to a Short Leg Syndrome

Ankylosing Spondylitis (Figure 3-40)

A 48-year-old preacher complained of severe bilaterally low back pain for 2 weeks. On questioning, he stated that he has had mild low back pain and hip pain for 3 years but he never sought medical care for this. There was no radiation of the pain into the lower extremities or increase of the pain on coughing and straining at the stool. He denied numbness, tingling, or weakness of the lower extremities.

Physical examination revealed tenderness of the lumbar spine and sacroiliac joints but sensation, power, and reflexes in the lower extremities were intact. SLR was negative bilaterally.

Laboratory examination revealed an elevated ESR and positive HLA B-27 antigen. x-Ray of the lumbosacral spine revealed moderate sclerosis of the sacroiliac joints and calcification of the anterior spinal ligament.

Treatment with NSAIDs and an exercise program produced moderate improvement, and he was able to resume his normal activities.

Differential Diagnosis

1. Reiter syndrome
2. Crohn disease
3. Psoriasis
4. Lumbar spondylosis
5. Herniated lumbar disc
6. Ochronosis

Discussion: Ninety percent of patients with this disorder are positive for HLA-B27 antigen. x-Ray findings may progress to marginal bulging syndesmophytes of the spine and poker spine in later stages. Plain films may be negative in the early stages, but an MRI may demonstrate inflammation and erosion of the S1 joints and vertebral bodies. Intra-articular corticosteroids may provide temporary relief, but TNF blocks such as etanercept may bring relief when NSAIDs fail.

Anterior view of lumbar spine

L1
L2
L3
L4
L5
Sacroiliac joint

Transverse view of lumbar spine

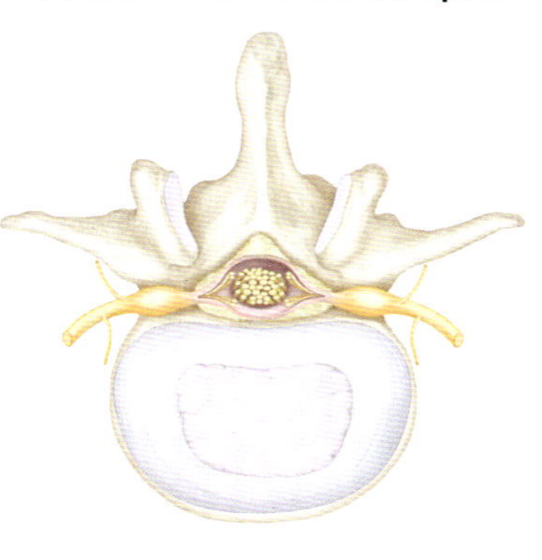

Sagittal view of lumbar spine

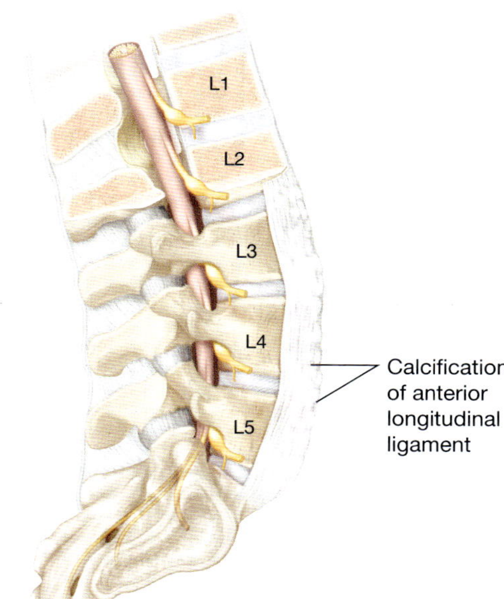

FIGURE 3-40: Ankylosing Spondylitis

Greater Trochanter Bursitis (Figure 3-41)

A 58-year-old white female slipped and fell on an icy sidewalk landing on her buttocks, 3 weeks prior to visiting her family doctor. She immediately had low back and left hip pain but no significant numbness, tingling, or weakness in her lower extremities. x-Rays of both hips were unremarkable. However, an x-ray of her lumbar spine showed narrowing of the disc spaces at L4-L5 and L5-S1 with associated osteoarthritic changes. She was treated conservatively with NSAIDs and muscle relaxants but failed to improve, so she was referred to a neurologist.

On examination, the neurologist found bilateral moderate erector spinae muscle spasm, but SLR and femoral stretch testing was negative bilaterally and there were no focal neurologic signs. However, she had a positive Patrick test on the left and exquisite tenderness of the left greater trochanter bursa.

A diagnosis of greater trochanter bursitis was made and confirmed by immediate relief of her hip and back pain by injecting the bursa with 5 cc of 2% Xylocaine without epinephrine and 60 mg of triamcinolone acetonide. For a complete description of the technique, the reader is referred to McNabb JW. *A Practical Guide to Joint and Soft Tissue Injections and Aspiration*. Philadelphia, PA: Lippincott Williams & Wilkins; 2005.

Differential Diagnosis

1. Herniated lumbar disc
2. Compression fracture of the lumbar spine
3. Fracture of the hip
4. Osteomyelitis of the hip
5. Osteoarthritis of the hip
6. Lumbar spondylosis

Discussion: Hip pathology is often misdiagnosed as radiculopathy caused by pathology in the lumbosacral spine. That is why a satisfactory examination of the patient with low back pain should always include a Patrick test. When in doubt, order x-ray of the hips along with x-rays of

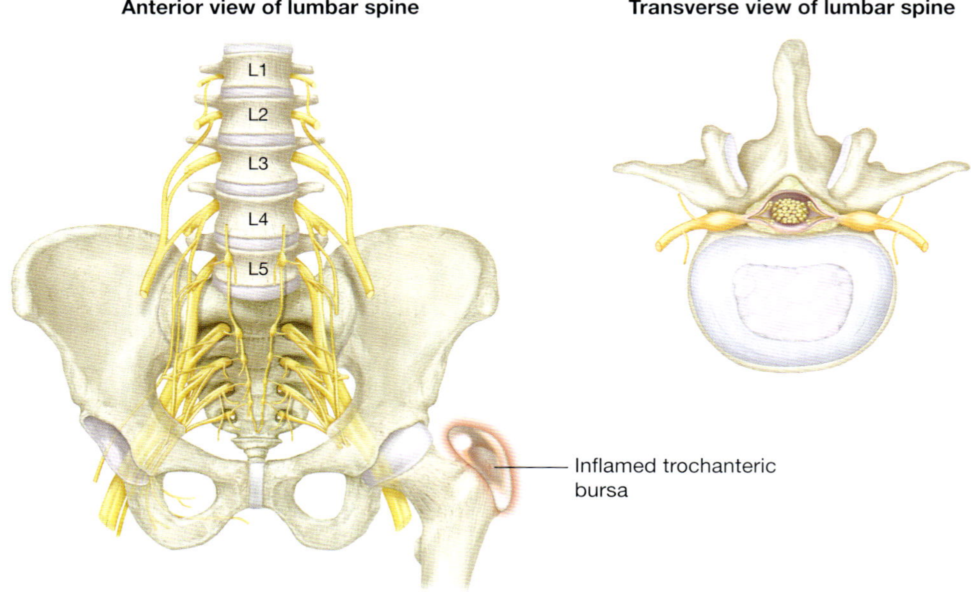

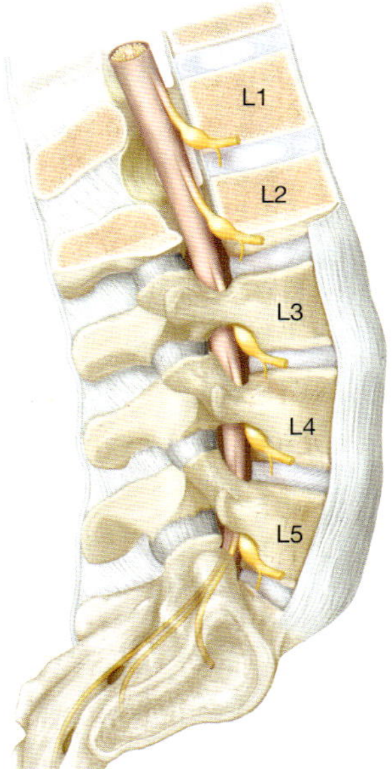

FIGURE 3-41: Greater Trochanter Bursitis

the lumbosacral spine. Another distinguishing feature is that pain due to osteoarthritis of the hip usually is in the groin while pain due to greater trochanter bursitis is always lateral to the hip joint.

REFERENCES

1. Bowdon G, et al. *Oxford Handbook of Orthopaedics and Trauma*. Oxford, UK: Oxford University Press; 2010:232.
2. Namdari S, et al. *Orthopedic Secrets*. 4th ed. London, NY: Elsevier Saunders; 2015.
3. Stauggard-Jones JA. *The Vital Psoas Muscles*. Chichester, England: Lutos Publishing; 2012:23.
4. Cherkin DC, et al. A comparison of physical therapy, chiropractic manipulation, and provision of an educational booklet for treatment of patients with low back pain. *N Engl J Med*. 1998;339:1021–1029.
5. Collins RD. One hundred consecutive epidural injections for back pain: therapeutic results and adverse side effects. *J Neurol Orthop Med Surg*. 1991;12:120–123.
6. Maf J. Worsening trends in the management and treatment of back pain. *JAMA Intern Med*. 2013;173:1573.
7. Laporte C, et al. MRI investigation of radiating pain in the lower limbs: value of an additional sequence dedicated to the lumbosacral plexus and pelvic girdle. *AJR Am J Roentgenol*. 2014;203:1280.

APPENDIX A

Illustrations of the Complete Routine Neurologic Examination

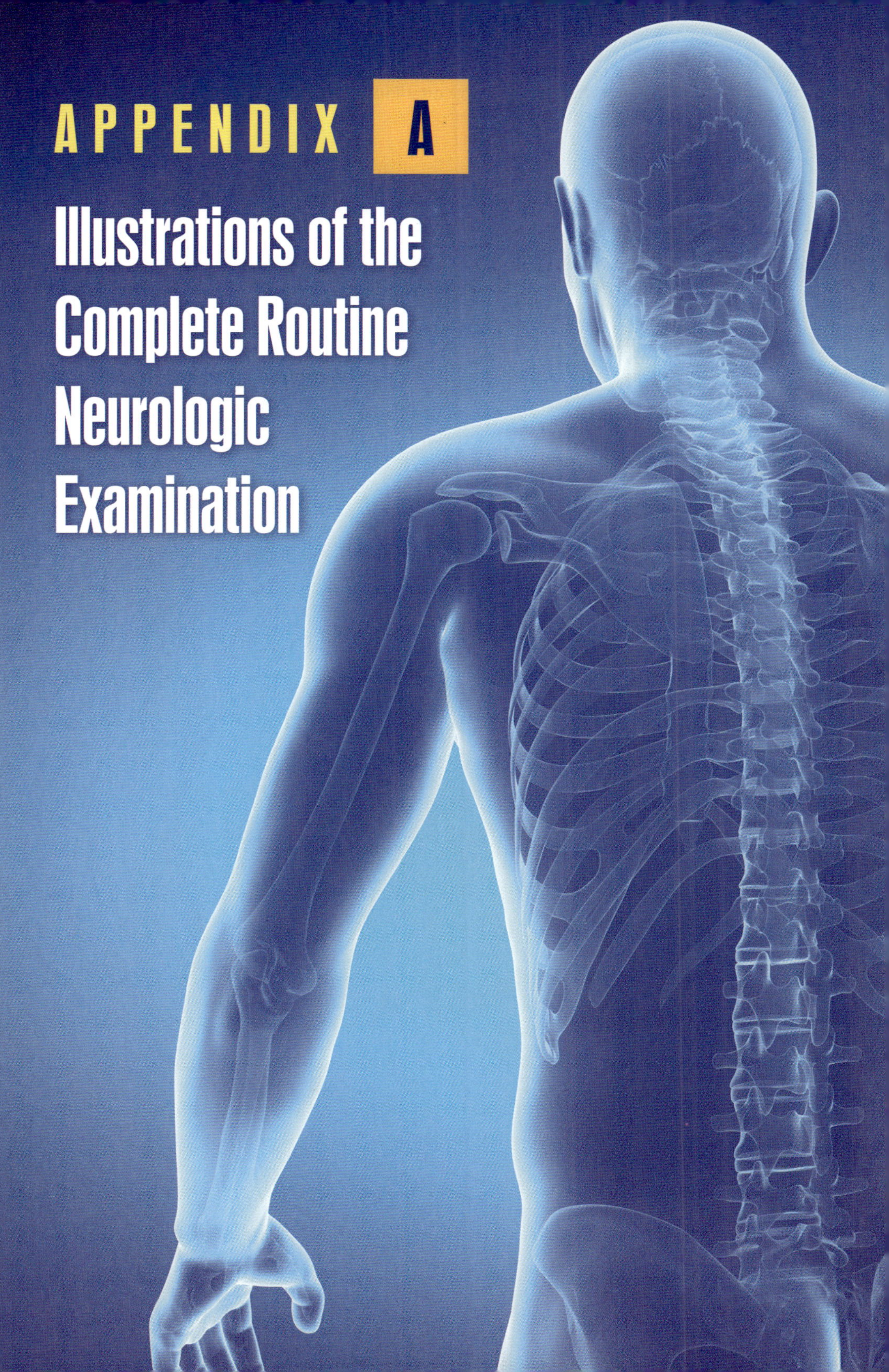

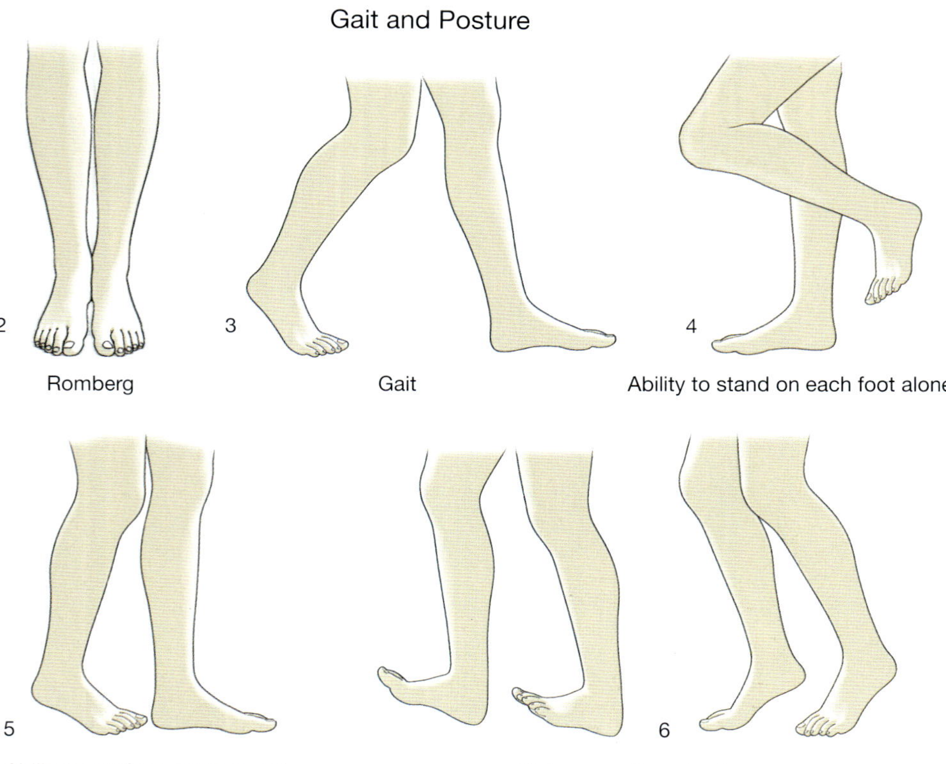

FIGURE A-1: From Collins RD. *Illustrated Manual of Neurologic Diagnosis*. 2nd ed. Philadelphia, PA: J.B. Lippincott Co.; 1982, with permission.

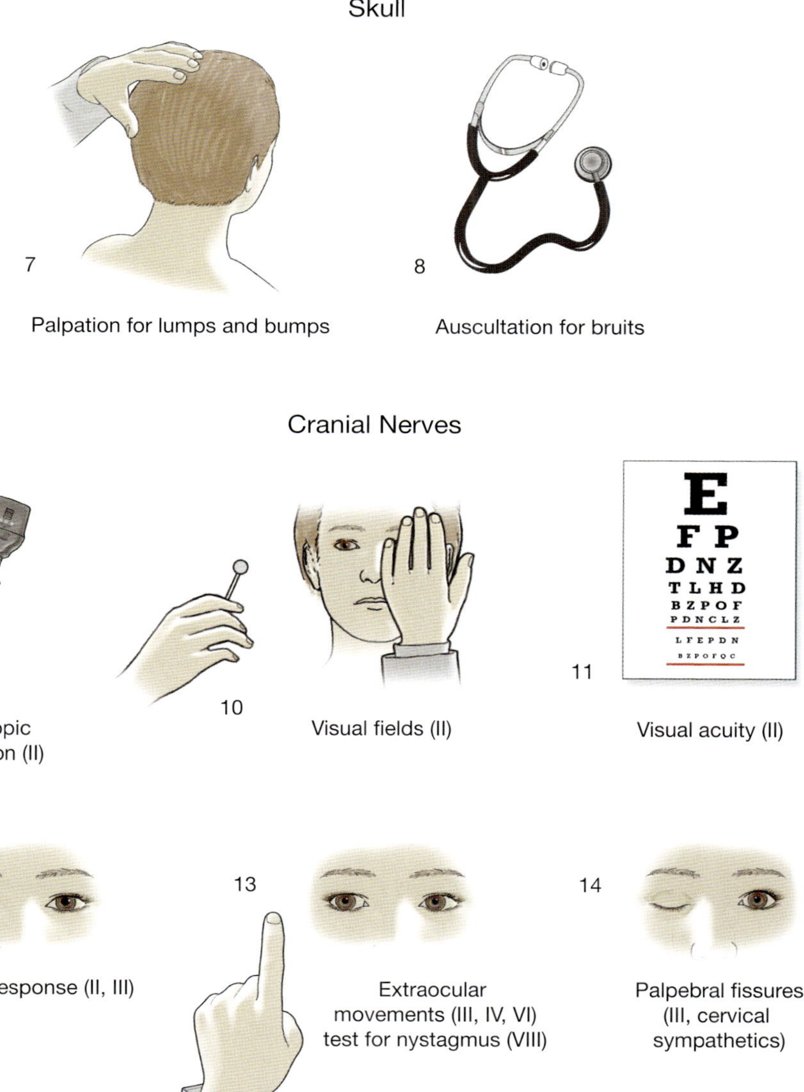

FIGURE A-2: From Collins RD. *Illustrated Manual of Neurologic Diagnosis*. 2nd ed. Philadelphia, PA: J.B. Lippincott Co.; 1982, with permission.

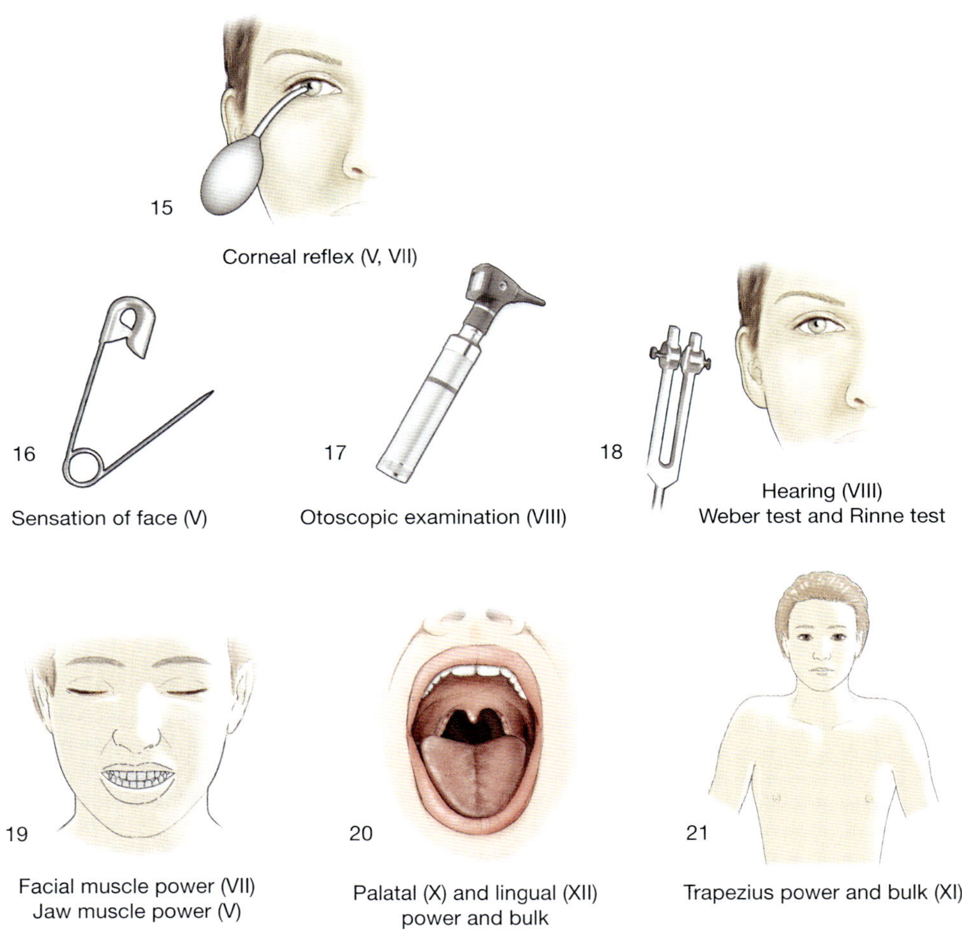

FIGURE A-3: From Collins RD. *Illustrated Manual of Neurologic Diagnosis*. 2nd ed. Philadelphia, PA: J.B. Lippincott Co.; 1982, with permission.

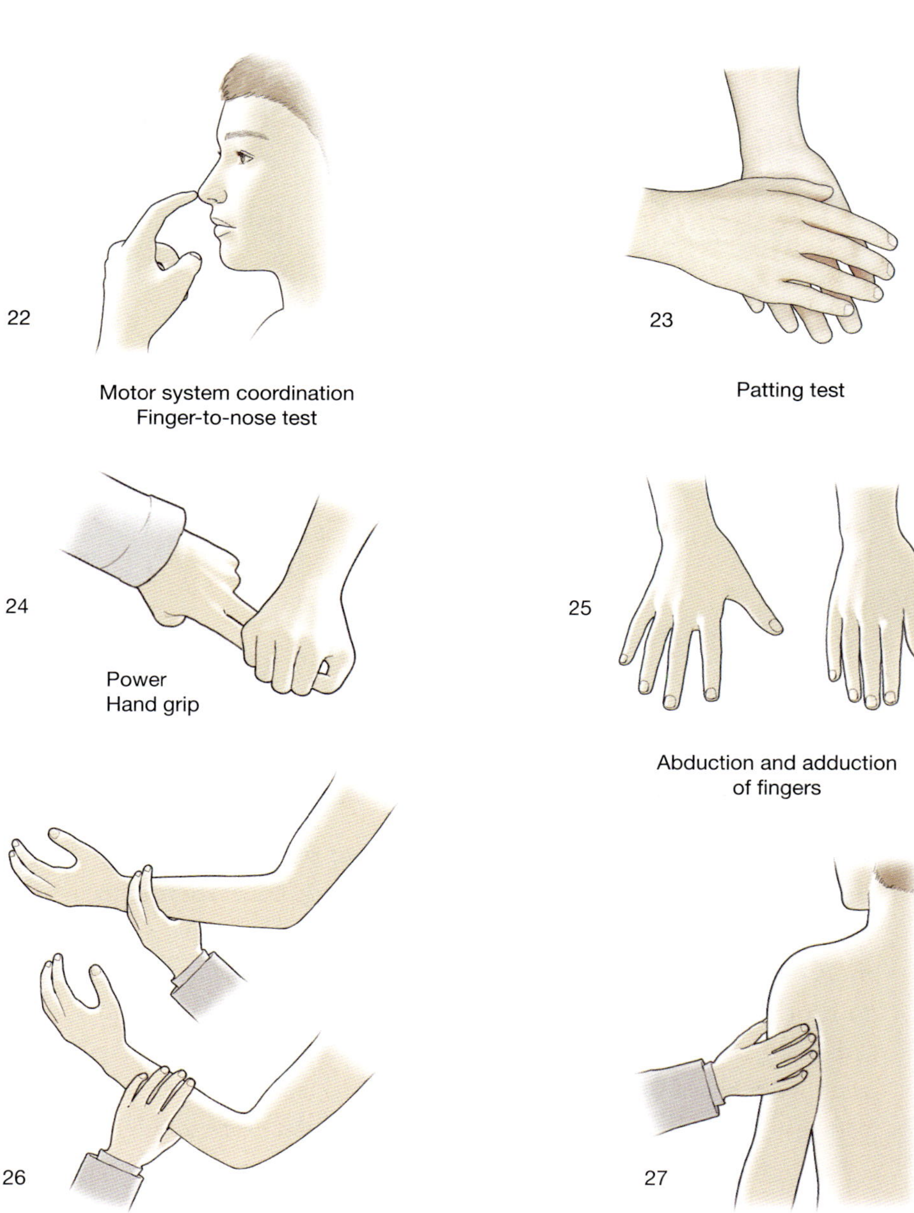

FIGURE A-4: From Collins RD. *Illustrated Manual of Neurologic Diagnosis*. 2nd ed. Philadelphia, PA: J.B. Lippincott Co.; 1982, with permission.

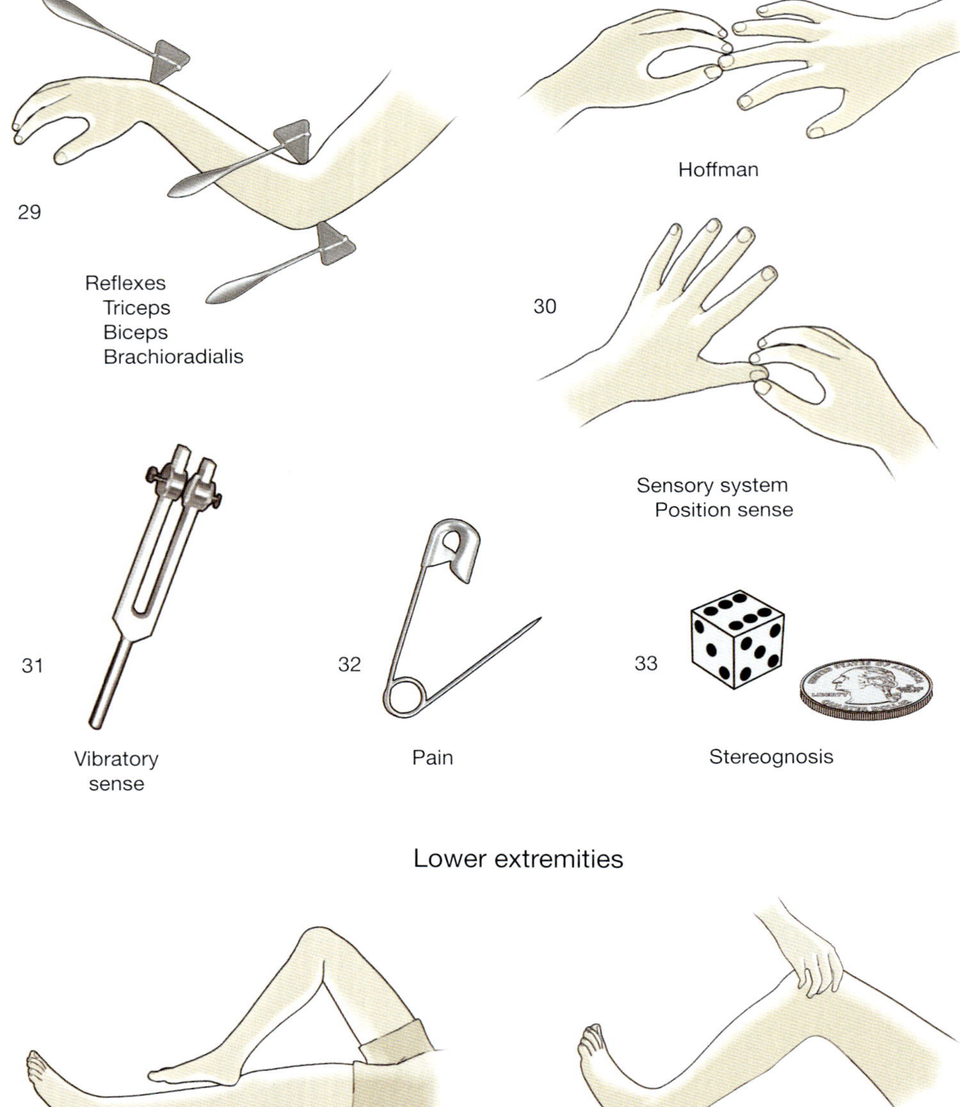

FIGURE A-5: From Collins RD. *Illustrated Manual of Neurologic Diagnosis*. 2nd ed. Philadelphia, PA: J.B. Lippincott Co.; 1982, with permission.

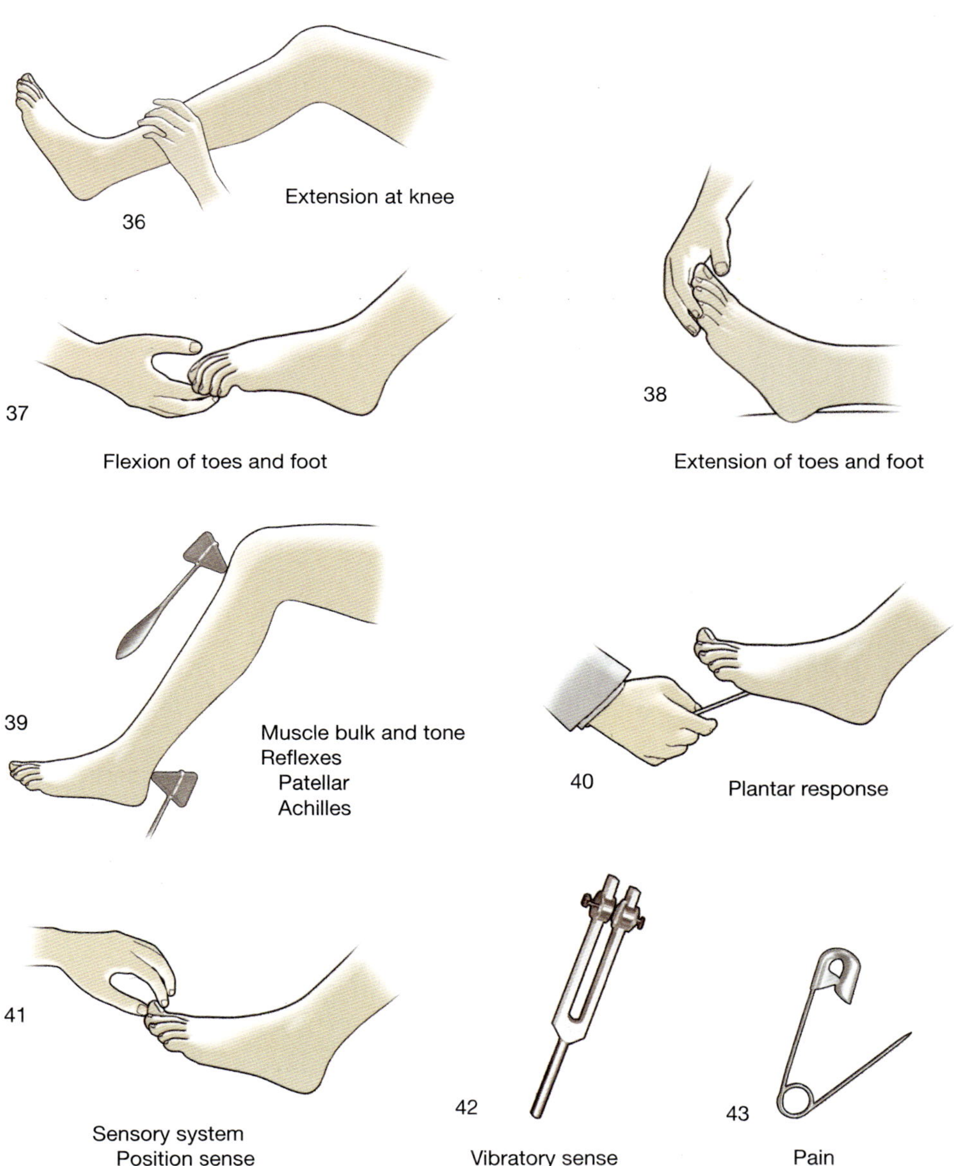

FIGURE A-6: From Collins RD. *Illustrated Manual of Neurologic Diagnosis*. 2nd ed. Philadelphia, PA: J.B. Lippincott Co.; 1982, with permission.

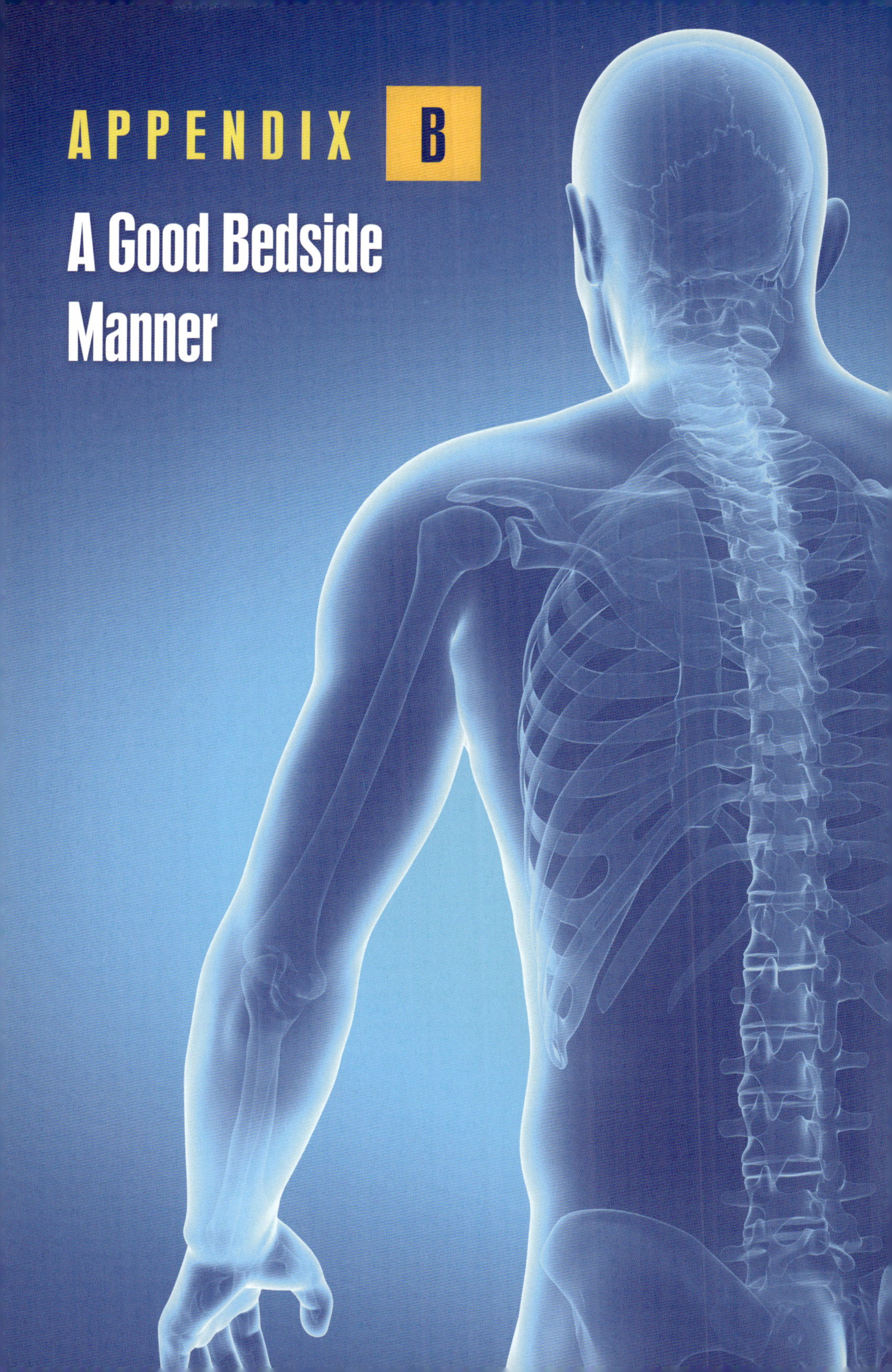

APPENDIX B

A Good Bedside Manner

After 50 years of practice, the author has developed several techniques that he would like to pass on to clinicians that may improve outcomes. He has also added the suggestions of several colleagues to this section.

1. Dress appropriately: If you want the trust and respect of your patient, you need to be clean and neat! More than that you should wear the traditional white coat. The white coat commands respect and is the symbol of our profession. Street clothes, a scrub suit or plaid shirt and jeans, just do not cut it even if you are clean. And wear a name tag, so they know who you are. It is also easy to turn a patient off with bad breath or B.O. The author keeps a bottle of mouth wash, Binaca, and deodorant handy to avoid this.
2. Greet the patient with a smile and a warm "Hello." Introduce yourself if it is the first visit. No matter how you feel, make the patient feel at home. No matter how many patients you've seen on any given day, make this one feel they are special. The author almost always greets the patient with a hand shake or hug as well. Many physicians need a personality transplant. Regardless of your basic demeanor, you can develop a warm and caring attitude if you try. Also, instead of getting right down to the medical problem at hand, ask them about their family, the weather, or some other nonmedical subject. (You will be surprised when some patient's only pain problem is due to a family fight.)
3. Listen to the patient: One of the greatest physicians who ever lived, William Osler said: "Listen to the patient and he/she will tell you the diagnosis." When you ask a question, give the patient time to answer. Establish eye contact! Do not interrupt, unless he or she starts to ramble on and on. Never act like you are in a hurry. Make the patient feel like he or she is the only patient you have.
4. Talk to the patient when you are doing the examination or procedure: Recently, the author visited Dr. Richard Benveniste, a periodontist in the Los Angeles area. Because he talked to his patient every step of the way, the procedure was much less painful. Fear was largely eliminated.

5. Be gentle with your examination: John Evans, FNP, points out that this is especially true of pediatric and elderly patients. He recommends starting by examining an area that is not painful and then move to the area that might be painful. He also recommends palpating a potentially tender area with the patient's fingers under his or hers.
6. Explain what you think is wrong: When you've finished your history and physical, do not just order a bunch of tests or write out a prescription and dismiss the patient. Explain what you think the problem is and what you are going to do about it. In addition to writing a prescription, you may need to write down specific instructions on what else to do so they do not forget them.
7. Go over laboratory and x-ray reports: Don't just tell the patient the results of their tests. Show them the reports. After all, the chart is theirs also, and they should be able to see everything on it. When giving bad news, always show compassion and leave the patient with hope. For example, "Yes, you've had a stroke but with 8 billion nerve cells, there's a good chance that other nerve cells will be able to take over for the ones you lost!"
8. Call the patient to see how he or she is doing: The author learned this from a highly respected chiropractor. If you've done a procedure, call the patient that evening or the next day to see how they are doing. That proves you care. The author also handles phone messages as soon as possible rather than waiting until the end of the day to handle them. By that time, the patient could be a lot worse (or dead) and the pharmacy may be closed.
9. Do not lose your temper: As physicians, we cannot have the luxury of a temper. It is the quickest way to loss the respect of your patient. You can be firm without being angry. If you are losing patience, it is time to refer the patient to a specialist or another primary care provider.
10. When in doubt, refer the patient out! Do not be afraid to admit you do not know what is going on. Call in a consultant. It is a lot cheaper than an MRI or a CT scan, and the patient will respect you for it.

11. Offer to pray with your patient: If you are a believer and you know your patient is too, this is an important part of treatment. You can include this question on your patient information inquiry. Back in the 90's, CBS News reported on a study that showed that people of faith recover more quickly following surgery.

APPENDIX C

Prescribing Opioids for Chronic Pain

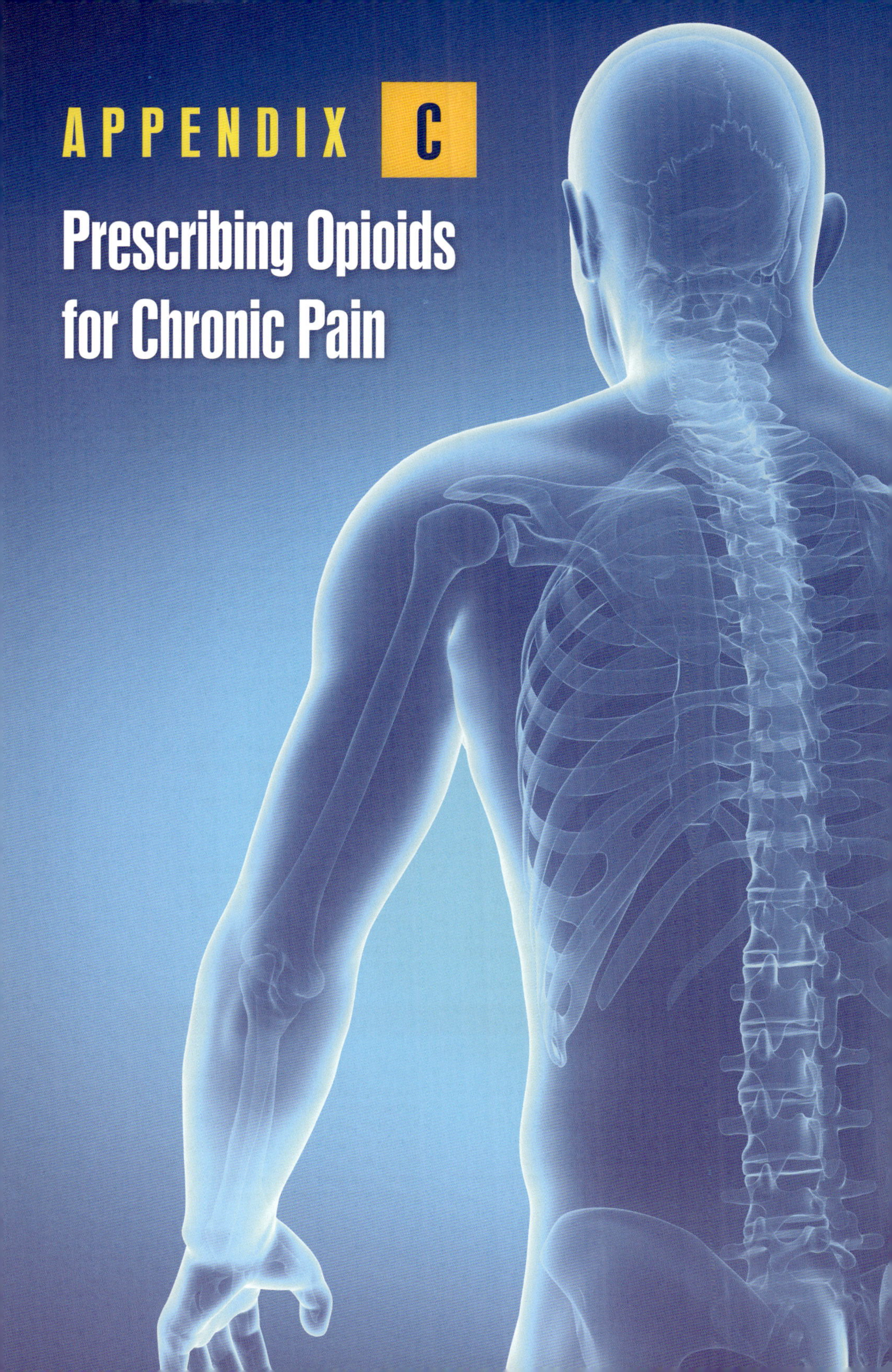

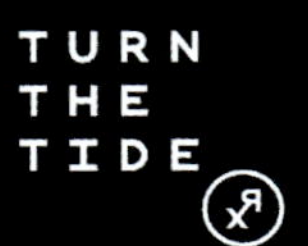

PRESCRIBING OPIOIDS FOR CHRONIC PAIN

ADAPTED FROM CDC GUIDELINE

Opioids can provide short-term benefits for moderate to severe pain. Scientific evidence is lacking for the benefits to treat chronic pain.

IN GENERAL, DO NOT PRESCRIBE OPIOIDS AS THE FIRST-LINE TREATMENT FOR CHRONIC PAIN (for adults 18+ with chronic pain > 3 months excluding active cancer, palliative, or end-of-life care).

BEFORE PRESCRIBING

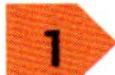

1 ASSESS PAIN & FUNCTION

Use a validated pain scale. Example: PEG scale where the score = average 3 individual question scores (30% improvement from baseline is clinically meaningful).

Q1: What number from 0 – 10 best describes your PAIN in the past week? (0 = "no pain", 10 = "worst you can imagine")

Q2: What number from 0 – 10 describes how, during the past week, pain has interfered with your ENJOYMENT OF LIFE? (0 = "not at all", 10 = "complete interference")

Q3: What number from 0 – 10 describes how, during the past week, pain has interfered with your GENERAL ACTIVITY? (0 = "not at all", 10 = "complete interference")

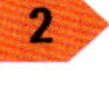

2 CONSIDER IF NON-OPIOID THERAPIES ARE APPROPRIATE

Such as: NSAIDs, TCAs, SNRIs, anti-convulsants, exercise or physical therapy, cognitive behavioral therapy.

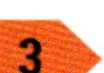

3 TALK TO PATIENTS ABOUT TREATMENT PLAN

- Set realistic goals for pain and function based on diagnosis.
- Discuss benefits, side effects, and risks (e.g., addiction, overdose).
- Set criteria for stopping or continuing opioid. Set criteria for regular progress assessment.
- Check patient understanding about treatment plan.

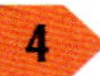

4 EVALUATE RISK OF HARM OR MISUSE. CHECK:

- Known risk factors: illegal drug use; prescription drug use for nonmedical reasons; history of substance use disorder or overdose; mental health conditions; sleep-disordered breathing.
- Prescription drug monitoring program data (if available) for opioids or benzodiazepines from other sources.
- Urine drug screen to confirm presence of prescribed substances and for undisclosed prescription drug or illicit substance use.
- Medication interactions. AVOID CONCURRENT OPIOID AND BENZODIAZEPINE USE WHENEVER POSSIBLE.

WHEN YOU PRESCRIBE

START LOW AND GO SLOW. IN GENERAL:

- Start with immediate-release (IR) opioids at the lowest dose for the shortest therapeutic duration. IR opioids are recommended over ER/LA products when starting opioids.
- Avoid ≥ 90 MME/day; consider specialist to support management of higher doses.
- If prescribing ≥ 50 MME/day, increase follow-up frequency; consider offering naloxone for overdose risk.
- For acute pain: prescribe < 3 day supply; more than 7 days will rarely be required.
- Counsel patients about safe storage and disposal of unused opioids.

See below for MME comparisons. For MME conversion factors and calulator, go to TurnTheTideRx.org/treatment.

50 MORPHINE MILLLIGRAM EQUIVALENTS (MME)/DAY:

- 50 mg of hydrocodone (10 tablets of hydrocodone/acetaminophen 5/300)
- 33 mg of oxycodone (~2 tablets of oxycodone sustained-release 15 mg)

90 MORPHINE MILLLIGRAM EQUIVALENTS (MME)/DAY:

- 90 mg of hydrocodone (18 tablets of hydrocodone/acetaminophen 5/300)
- 60 mg of oxycodone (4 tablets of oxycodone sustained-release 15 mg)

AFTER INITIATION OF OPIOID THERAPY

ASSESS, TAILOR & TAPER

- Reassess benefits/risks within 1–4 weeks after initial assessment.
- Assess pain and function and compare results to baseline. Schedule reassessment at regular intervals (≤ 3 months).
- Continue opioids only after confirming clinically meaningful improvements in pain and function without significant risks or harm.
- If over-sedation or overdose risk, then taper. Example taper plan: 10% decrease in original dose per week or month. Consider psychosocial support.
- Tailor taper rates individually to patients and monitor for withdrawal symptoms.

TREATING OVERDOSE & ADDICTION

- Screen for opioid use disorder (e.g., difficulty controlling use; see DSM-5 criteria). If yes, treat with medication-assisted treatment (MAT). MAT combines behavioral therapy with medications like methadone, buprenorphine, and naltrexone. Refer to findtreatment.samhsa.gov. Additional resources at TurnTheTideRx.org/treatment and www.hhs.gov/opioids.
- Learn about medication-assisted treatment (MAT) and apply to be a MAT provider at www.samhsa.gov/medication-assisted-treatment.
- Consider offering naloxone if high risk for overdose: history of overdose or substance use disorder, higher opioid dosage (≥ 50 MME/day), concurrent benzodiazepine use.

ADDITIONAL RESOURCES

CDC GUIDELINE FOR PRESCRIBING OPIOIDS FOR CHRONIC PAIN: www.cdc.gov/drugoverdose/prescribing/guideline.html

SAMHSA POCKET GUIDE FOR MEDICATION-ASSISTED TREATMENT (MAT): store.samhsa.gov/MATguide

NIDAMED: www.drugabuse.gov/nidamed-medical-health-professionals

ENROLL IN MEDICARE: go.cms.gov/pecos
Most prescribers will be required to enroll or validly opt out of Medicare for their prescriptions for Medicare patients to be covered. Delay may prevent patient access to medications.

JOIN THE MOVEMENT

of health care practitioners committed to ending the opioid crisis at TurnTheTideRx.org.

TURN THE TIDE

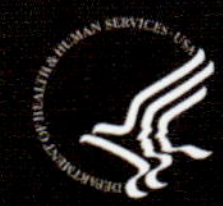

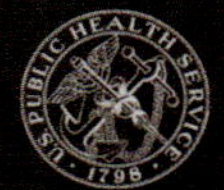

The Office of the Surgeon General

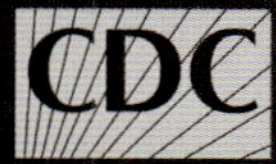

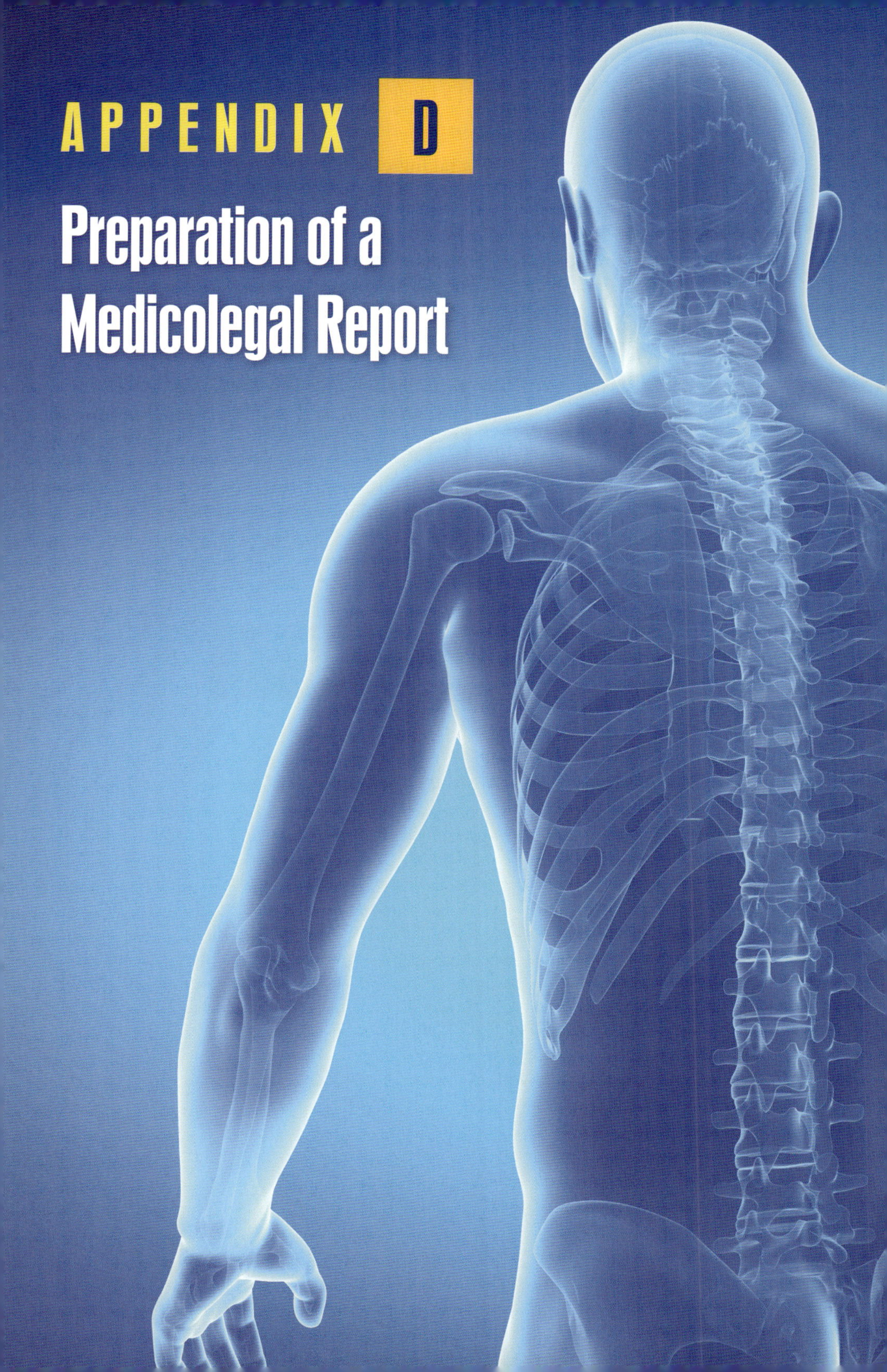

APPENDIX D

Preparation of a Medicolegal Report

As a primary care provider who is taking care of patients with neck and back pain, you will no doubt be asked to prepare a medicolegal report from time to time as many of these patients have been in an accident of some kind that caused or aggravated their pain. Having prepared thousands of these reports, I feel, I must share my experiences with you. You can readily see from Table D-1, you cannot just write or dictate a report based on your history, physical, diagnosis, and treatment or SOAP notes. What follows is a detailed discussion of each of the topics in Table D-1, and we will end this discussion by a sample medicolegal report of a real patient, whose identity will not be disclosed for obvious reasons.

1. *Chief Complaint(s)*: This is not much different than the development of chief complaint(s) you have made on nonaccident victims, but you need to indicate whether they began on the date of the accident or

TABLE D-1

Outline of a Medicolegal Report

1. Chief Complaint(s)
2. History of the Accident
3. What Happened to the Patient During the Accident?
4. Initial Medical Care
5. Review of Systems
6. Past History
7. Job Description
8. Review of Medical Records
9. Physical Examination
10. Impression or Diagnosis
11. Causation
12. Diagnostic Workup
13. Treatment
14. Prognosis
15. Disability
16. Future Medical Care

existed prior to the accident but were aggravated by the accident. Be sure to gauge the intensity of the pain on a scale of 1 to 10 and how it interferes with their activities of daily living or job on a scale of 1 to 10.

2. *History of Accident*: If this is work related, what was the patient doing at the onset of the pain (bending, stooping, lifting a heavy object, etc.) or if it was a motor vehicle accident (MVA), was the car the patient was in rear-ended, T-boned, or in a head-on collision, etc. Have the patient draw a picture of the accident if possible. Also, where was the patient sitting in the car (driver, front or back seat passenger).
3. *What Happened to the Patient During the Accident?* Did he or she strike her head and lose consciousness or jerk his or her head or whole body back and forth or sideways, etc.? What symptoms were experienced immediately after the accident? If none of the symptoms in the chief complaint appeared right after the accident, when did they begin?
4. *Initial Medical Care*: Did the patient go to the emergency room or see another medical professional immediately? What was the immediate diagnosis and treatment and were imaging studies done? If so, what were the results?
5. *Review of Systems*: Many times, the patient will forget some symptoms that were caused by the accident, so a careful review of systems is important.
6. *Past History*: Here, it is important to find out if the patient has experienced a previous work-related accident or MVA that may have been associated with the same complaints. You need to know if the complaints experienced in previous accidents had completely cleared up or were still lingering at the time of the new accident. Also, whether the complaints associated with this accident were an aggravation of a preexisting medical condition (osteoarthritis, hypertension, congestive heart failure, etc.). You may find that this patient has "compensationitis" or is deliberately accident prone.

7. *Job Description*: This is usual only necessary in workman's compensation reports. You need this so you can address how the injury will affect their ability to perform their job and what work restriction applies.
8. *Review of Medical Records*: Frequently, the patient will have been seen by other doctors or visited the emergency room and even been hospitalized. You need to get these records and comment on each of them in your report. If they are totally unrelated to the accident, so state that fact. X-rays, CT scans, MRIs, and positive laboratory tests especially need to be reviewed and commented on.
9. *Your Physical Examination*: Here, you only need to list the positive findings. There is no need to try to impress the attorney with your medical acumen and the thoroughness of your examination! Why make the report longer than necessary?
10. *Impression or Diagnosis*: Make a list of all the conditions beginning with those that are a direct result of the accident and follow them with the conditions that were aggravated by the accident. It is optional whether you mention conditions here that are not related to the accident.
11. *Causation*: If it is not clear in your discussion under "Impression or Diagnosis" that you related each condition to the accident and specified the date you need to do that here. For example, "It is clear that this patient suffered a flexion-extension injury as a result of the accident of (date), resulting in a cervical sprain and aggravation of a pre-existing cervical spondylosis."
12. *Diagnostic Workup*: Here, you would list the orders for laboratory, x-rays, CT scans, MRIs, and other special diagnostic procedures you are planning. In your final report, you would discuss the results of these especially if they are positive and confirm your clinical impression.
13. *Treatment*: Here, you would list the various categories of drugs you will prescribe, physiotherapy or chiropractic treatment you recommend, and whether you feel the patient needs immediate surgery. You may feel a consult with an anesthesiologist is worthwhile for nerve blocks

or epidural injections. Alternatively, mention if an orthopedic or neurosurgical consult is necessary.

14. *Prognosis*: You will address the chances of a full recovery here. If you think that is not likely, so state it.
15. *Disability*: You may not be able to determine this on your initial evaluation because the patient may not have had the benefit of medical or surgical treatment at that point. Still you should address the subject. For example, "I am not able to address disability at this time because the patient has not had the benefit of treatment." Another example, "At this time, this patient is temporarily partially disabled and is restricted from frequent stooping or bending or lifting over 25 pounds!"

    In your final report, you should make a statement regarding permanent disability. For example, "This patient is permanent and stationary at this time and is left with a permanent partial disability requiring a restriction to light duty. Therefore, he is unable to continue his job stocking grocery stores and needs retrained for a job requiring only sedentary work."
16. *Future Medical Care*: Frequently, a patient whose condition has become permanent and stationary will need ongoing medical treatment for his or her condition. So, you must state this in your report. For example, "This patient will require 8–10 visits a year to his physician for evaluation and refilling his analgesic medications as well as an occasional series of physiotherapy treatments 3 times a week for 4–6 weeks." Some patients may need future surgery. For example, "This patient is not a candidate for a lumbar laminectomy at this time, but if in the future his radiculopathy causes weakness or atrophy of the muscles in his right leg or intractable pain which cannot be managed by anti-inflammatory agents, muscle relaxants or narcotics, surgery will be required."

What follows are examples of preliminary and final medicolegal reports:

Sample Initial Medicolegal Report

Attorney John Smith
Court Street
Pensacola, FL 32503
RE: Jane Doe

Dear Attorney Smith,

I saw Jane Doe in my office on July 27, 2009 at which time she gave the following history:

On June 21, 2009, her vehicle was stopped because the one in front of her was making a left turn and suddenly, a third vehicle, a Pontiac sedan, rammed into the back of her car forcing it into the vehicle in front. Her vehicle was totaled while the other one in front of her is reported to have sustained approximately $6,000.00 worth of damage.

She was riding in the back seat and her head was thrown forward by the impact and her head struck the front seat and she sustained a large knot on her forehead. She was confused immediately after the accident but denies retrograde amnesia.

She was taken to the Sacred Heart Emergency Room where she was examined and a CT scan ordered. After the evaluation was complete, she was told she had a concussion and was instructed to follow-up with her family physician.

Present Complaints

Since the accident, she has been forgetful. For example, she cannot remember her password when she is trying to get into her computer. She frequently misplaces things at home.

She is only getting 5 hours of sleep at night because her sleep is frequently interrupted. She also is irritable since the accident. She developed headache and neck and back pain, and these symptoms have continued almost constantly since.

Also, following the accident, she developed pain in her clavicles and anterior chest for the first 2 weeks, but these symptoms have cleared.

The neck pain is located in the suboccipital area bilaterally and radiates down both arms more on the left. She denies having this pain prior to the accident. Lately, it is constant. It is, however, not increased by coughing or sneezing.

The back pain is bilateral, posterior, and intermittent but at least 1 to 2 hours a day. Initially, it was increased by coughing and sneezing but not now. It does not radiate into the extremities.

The headache is located in the temples, occipital areas, and behind the eyes. It occurs at least 2 to 3 hours daily and will go away completely only to return. There is no associated nausea or vomiting, but she had a poor appetite for the first 2 weeks after the accident. There is no aura to the headaches. Immediately after the accident, her eyes were very sensitive to light. She never had these headaches prior to the accident. She developed blurred vision immediately after the accident and that has continued to the present. She denies any other symptomatology related to the accident.

Past History

The only time she has been hospitalized was for pregnancy and delivery. She denies any serious illnesses. She had a laparoscopy for infertility but no other surgery.

She was in a car accident in 1998 when she was a passenger in the right front seat and another car rammed her car on the front right side. She denies having sustained a concussion from that accident but did develop low back pain that subsequently cleared.

Following the accident of June 21, 2009, she began treatment with a chiropractor. He performed x-rays of the neck and low back and told her there were torn ligaments and twisted pelvis but no fracture or herniated disc evident.

She denies allergies or any communicable diseases other than chicken pox. She is presently not on any medication, although the Sacred Heart ER did give her analgesics and muscle relaxants, but she hesitates to take these because they seem to interfere with her job. She is back to work for the past 2 weeks.

Family History

Her father died of a heart condition. Her mother is still alive at 78 years old but has diabetes and hypertension.

Review of Systems

She had an immediate menstrual period after the accident, which was unexpected because she had just finished one prior to the accident. Otherwise, her review of systems is remarkably negative. The egg-sized lump on her forehead has subsided, but the forehead is still tender.

Review of Records

There are no records accompanying this patient.

Neurologic Examination

Neurologic examination today revealed the following positive findings

1. Tender slightly swollen forehead bilaterally.
2. Tender suboccipital area bilaterally.
3. She has 2+ splenius capitis and trapezius muscle spasm bilaterally.
4. Erector spinae muscle spasm bilaterally.
5. Pupils slightly dilated but react sluggishly to light and accommodation. Her vision is 20/40 for distance in the left eye and 20/50 in the right. She does not recall having this problem prior to the accident. Otherwise, the cranial nerves are intact, and there is symmetrical power, coordination, reflexes, and sensation on all four extremities. There are no pathologic reflexes. Gait and station are intact. Mental status is physiologic.

Impression

I believe this lady suffered a concussion and cervical and lumbar extension–flexion injury as a result of the accident of June 21, 2009, and now is left with a postconcussion syndrome, a cervical sprain, and a lumbosacral sprain.

Recommendation

At this time, I can only recommend symptomatic treatment in the form of analgesics, NSAIDs, and muscle relaxants, but she is reluctant to take these because of her job.

She should continue physiotherapy with her chiropractor. At this time, I do not recommend imaging studies, but they may be necessary in the future if her symptoms persist. I would like to get an EEG prior to her discharge from my care, however. She should be seen by an ophthalmologist or optometrist regarding her visual acuity.

Disability Status

She is temporarily partially disabled as a result of the accident of June 21, 2009, with a work restriction limiting lifting to no more than 25 pounds and no stooping or bending at this time.

I will follow her with bi-weekly visits until she is permanent and stationary.

Sincerely,

R. Douglas Collins, MD, FACP
Neurologist & Internist

Sample Final Medicolegal Report

Attorney John Smith
Court Street
Pensacola, FL 32503
RE: Jane Doe

Dear Attorney Smith,

I saw Jane Doe in my office on January 13, 2010, for a final evaluation at which time she stated the following:

Since her last visit, she had no headaches, nausea, vomiting, loss of consciousness, or other neurologic symptomatology except neck and back pain. However, she continues with ocular difficulties, and the iritis she experienced after the accident has developed in her right eye as well as her left. She never had iritis in the eye prior to the accident of June 21, 2009.

Her ophthalmologist has referred her to a rheumatologist who agrees with me that her iritis with a reasonable degree of medical certainty is the result of this accident.

Furthermore, she continues to experience suboccipital and cervical pain, which is a 4 on a scale of 1 to 10, and lumbar pain, which is a 3 on a scale of 1 to 10 becoming 9 on a scale of 1 to 10 on any significant activity.

Neurologic Examination

Neurologic examination today revealed the following positive findings

1. Her right pupil is oval and slightly dilated compared to the left but reacts to light and accommodation.
2. Right optic disc is pale, but there is no papilledema.
3. She has 3+ trapezius and splenius capitis muscle spasm bilaterally.
4. Range of motion of her C-spine is limited to 25 degrees lateral bending to the right and 30 degrees left with normal being 50 degrees.
5. She has 4+ sacrospinalis muscle spasm on the left without limitation of motion.

Final Impression

1. Concussion without evidence of postconcussion syndrome caused by the accident of June 21, 2009.
2. Autoimmune iritis of the left eye precipitated by the accident of June 21, 2009.
3. Precipitation of autoimmune iritis in the right eye by the accident of June 21, 2009.
4. Cervical sprain as a result of the accident of June 21, 2009.
5. Lumbosacral sprain as a result of the accident of June 21, 2009.

Disability

At this time, Ms. Doe is permanent and stationary. I believe she has recovered fully from her concussion, but because of the autoimmune iritis in the left eye and right eye, she will have a permanent partial disability related to the accident of June 21, 2009. She is able to continue with her employment as a clerk at the Social Security Office, but this may become impossible in the future.

Furthermore, I believe she will be left with a permanent partial disability as a result of her cervical and lumbar sprain. Once again, this has not interfered with her job at the Social Security Office. However, she requires a restriction of no lifting over 25 pounds and limited stooping and bending because of her cervical and lumbar sprains.

Future Medical Care

From a neurologic stand point, I would recommend a wake and sleep EEG in 1 year, and she should report any episodes of strange behavior or loss of consciousness to her family doctor immediately. Also, she may require treatment with analgesics, muscle relaxants, and chiropractic or physiotherapy from time to time because of her cervical and lumbar sprains.

Prognosis

It is my opinion that she has a five times greater than normal chance of developing epilepsy in the future as a result of the accident of June 21, 2009.

Sincerely,

R. Douglas Collins, MD, FACP
Neurologist

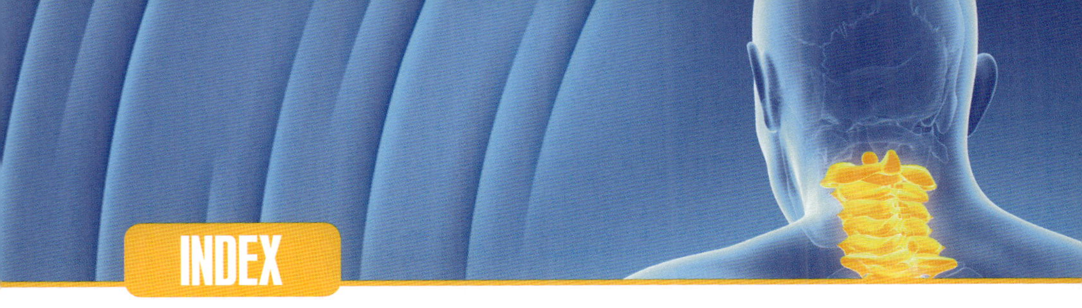

INDEX

Note: Page numbers followed by *f* indicate figures; page numbers followed by *t* indicate tables.

M

N